TEACHING NUTRITION

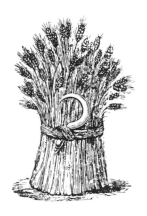

TEACHING
NUTRITION
A Review of
Programs and
Research

Edited by
Joanne P. Nestor and Judith A. Glotzer

Abt Books   Cambridge, Massachusetts

Reissued by arrangement with
University Press of America, Inc.
4720 Boston Way
Lanham, MD 20706

Library of Congress Cataloging in Publication Data
Main entry under title:

Teaching nutrition.

Includes bibliographies and index.
Contents: A conceptual framework for individual nutrition influences, responses, and impacts / by Joanne P. Nestor — Evaluation of nutrition education / by Judy K. Brun — Teaching training in nutrition education / by Joanne P. Nestor — [etc.]
1. Nutrition—Study and teaching. I. Nestor, Joanne P., 1949-
II. Glotzer, Judith A., 1947-
TX364.T42   641.1'07'1   81-66087
ISBN 0-89011-559-1   AACR2

Printed in the United States of America

Book and cover design by: Martha Scotford Lange

CONTENTS

1

A Conceptual Framework for Individual Nutrition

Joanne P. Nestor

2

Evaluation of Nutrition Education: A Review

Judy K. Brun

3

Teacher Training in Nutrition Education

Joanne P. Nestor

4

Education and Training for School Food Service Personnel

Allene G. Vaden

5

Preschool Nutrition Education

Christine Olson and Jill Randell

6

Kindergarten Through Sixth Grade Nutrition Education

Isobel Contento

7
Secondary School Nutrition Education
Martha L. Plass and Martha C. Mapes

Appendices

ACKNOWLEDGMENTS

Many organizations and individuals have helped to make this book possible. We are indebted to Audrey Maretzki and Barbara Fontana of the U.S. Department of Agriculture, Food and Nutrition Service, for their support of the project upon which this document is based, and particularly for helping us identify and recruit the contributors and secure the cooperation of the Food and Nutrition Information Center.

At Abt Associates Inc., Thomas Ferb directed the project, and staff nutritionists Mary Kay Fox, Ellen Glovsky, and Patricia Granahan contributed to the literature search. David Napior assisted in developing the conceptual framework presented in Chapter One and in recruiting consultants. Robert Dentler and Marian Zeitlin reviewed early drafts and provided constructive suggestions for additions and revisions. Thomas Ferb, Robert Dentler, and Robert Erwin encouraged and supported us in our efforts to transform the original document into this book. Margaret Anthony provided patient and reliable assistance in production of the manuscript.

Special thanks are due to friends and family for their support: Valerie, Linda and Phil, Jim and Joanne, Andrew, Claire, and Rose.

INTRODUCTION

Public investment in nutrition education is justified by the public's need to make nutritionally valid food choices. As the food supply grows more complex and expensive, consumer skills become vital. Many of the major health problems of the past have been conquered through improved standards of living and medical care. Contagious diseases no longer figure among the major causes of death in the United States. Instead, degenerative diseases, many of which are related to nutrition, now take a heavy toll in lives and consume a large proportion of the health care budget. Responsibility for prevention of these health problems and even for remedies cannot be placed on doctors or other professionals, for the problems are rooted in the daily choices everyone makes about what to eat. Therefore, the public must be able and willing to take responsibility for its own nutritional well-being. Nutrition education is the primary method for improving nutrition knowledge, attitudes, and behavior, and since children in school are in the process of acquiring knowledge and lifetime habits, the school is a logical focus for public nutrition education. Until very recently, however, school programs in nutrition education were few and their impact small.

The Nutrition Education and Training Program

The Nutrition Education and Training (NET) Program was established in 1977 by PL 95–166, an amendment to the 1966 Child Nutrition Act. Its legislated purpose is "to encourage effective dissemination of scientifically valid information to children participating or eligible to participate in school lunch and related child nutrition programs." NET funds are distributed through state education agencies to local schools and districts for use in training teachers and school food service personnel and in conducting nutrition education activities that fully utilize both the school food service facilities and the classroom.

Because of the innovative nature of the program and the need for information on the program's development, the U.S. Department of Agriculture (USDA) initiated an evaluation of the program, to be conducted during its third year of operation. That evaluation is now being conducted by Abt Associates Inc. of Cambridge, Massachusetts, and some preliminary results are cited in this report (Ferb 1980).

A preliminary task in a project evaluation is to review existing programs and research literature. As the Abt Associates researchers began to review the literature on nutrition education, they realized that it is unlike that of many other fields. Consensus has not been reached on evaluation measures or methodologies; indeed, much of the literature is anecdotal. There is little cross-referencing among articles—evidence of the lack of agreement on principles. Definitions and methodologies are unclear. The only relevant journal (the *Journal of Nutrition Education*) has been in existence for only ten years and is a quarterly publication. Finally, no review of the literature has been published since Whitehead's 1973 review of work to 1970, which did not focus on children. It was evident that a thorough review of the literature relevant to NET was required, not only for the sake of the current project, but also to serve as a tool for NET personnel and other nutrition educators, researchers, and planners who are designing or assessing nutrition programs. With the consent and advice of the Abt NET Evaluation Project's advisors at the USDA, an expanded effort was undertaken, and experts in the field were asked to contribute to it.

Because this document is an outgrowth of the NET Program, topics are limited to those relevant to NET: the training of food service personnel and teachers, and the state of in-school nutrition education for children through high school age. Because of the striking need for refinement and development of evaluation procedures, a section specific to this need is also included. Almost all the knowledge we have of nutrition education is based on small-scale studies with minimally adequate evaluation components and little or no reference to large-scale issues. Many factors outside of school-based nutrition education influence children's nutrition behavior and status; these factors must not be overlooked. Therefore, we adopted a nutrition intake model developed by Abt staff for another project. We present this model first to serve as a framework for the subsequent sections of the book.

The format selected has two drawbacks, which we recognize but had to accept because of the nature of the work. First, there is no separate section on materials and curricula; rather, these are discussed in the sections dealing with specific target groups. Materials and curricula cannot stand alone: someone must use them, and their impact on their audiences must be evaluated. Furthermore, catalogs of materials and curricula are already available from several nutrition agencies and organizations.

The second problem with this format is that it masks any cooperation between training programs for teachers and those for food service personnel. Such cooperation is indeed one of the major goals of the NET Program and has been demonstrated to improve the effect of nutrition education, but most of the literature available addresses only one of the two groups, so cooperative efforts are described in both the relevant sections.

Several other topics were considered for inclusion in this book but were omitted because of the need to focus on NET participants and goals. These topics, which are no less relevant to children's nutrition status and are as sorely in need of reviewing as the topics included, are parent education, mass media, institutional education programs (for example, hospital programs), and other federal food programs affecting children (for example, the Special Supplemental Food Program for Women, Infants, and Children; and Food Stamps).

Summary of Findings

One common thread running through all the papers is that the state of the art of nutrition education is still in its infancy; it is indeed an art rather than a science. Across the broad range of nutrition education activities, one cannot easily identify alternative theoretical approaches. Since the approaches to behavioral change have not been well articulated in the literature, there seems to have been very little theory development. Theory in nutrition education is implicit, as it is in many formative sciences operating in applied settings. The field seems to be driven more by practical and economic concerns related to school feeding programs than by sound theory.

Goals and techniques have changed little in several decades. Although numerous sets of nutrition goals and guidelines based on expert opinions have been published since the 1960s, most training programs and curricula do not take them into account. Nor do most recognize the many factors other than nutrition knowledge which influence behavior: students are influenced by peers, television, and family; teachers and food service personnel are influenced by conflicting demands and attitudes. Research and evaluation of projects are hampered by several problems, resulting in a body of information of uncertain quality and limited generalizability. Among the problems are lack of a consensus on desirable behaviors and attitudes and on necessary knowledge; lack of recognition of the complexity of the interrelationships among knowledge, attitudes, and behaviors; development of new instrumentation for almost every study, hindering generalizability; and lack of the time, money, and skilled personnel required for research and evaluation.

These problems are most evident in the area of behavioral change: we lack well-defined and justified statements of the behavioral changes that nutrition education should produce. Also lacking are measures that take into account the many factors contributing to children's food choices. Evaluation is tacked on as an afterthought to many programs or is included only as a concession to sponsors' requirements for accountability, rendering it useless for general program development.

The increasing demand for accountability of publicly funded programs, including NET projects, is contributing to a recent trend toward refinement of project evaluation techniques and recognition of the wide variety of factors that influence food-related behavior. In order to benefit from this trend, we need to improve our communications systems and provide greater access to unpublished materials. Long-term studies are needed not only to assess behavioral outcomes more effectively, but also to examine the ultimate effects on children of nutrition programs for teachers and food service personnel.

Conceptual Framework. Most of the programs encountered gave little or no recognition of their relationship to the student's overall nutrition environment. In-school programs, in particular, gave little attention to the effects on students of family, income, cultural beliefs, attitudes and practices regarding food, physiological food needs, and real-world eating options. Instead, most focused on in-school experiences, despite statements of broader purposes. Therefore, in the interest of providing a perspective on school-based nutrition and a framework for discussing its elements, Chapter One provides a model of the student's entire immediate nutrition environment, external and internal. The model is intended not to illustrate causal relationships, few of which have been conclusively established, but rather to present a context within which information and relationships about children's nutrition can be discussed.

Evaluation.   A major obstacle to program design and evaluation is the need for clarification of the purposes of nutrition education and of the terminology used. The necessary instrumentation cannot be developed without consensus on the definitions of variables. Even if this consensus existed, however, not all nutrition educators could be expected to have the skills or time to evaluate programs on a major scale; smaller but continuous evaluation procedures can provide the necessary feedback for program improvement and decision making.

Meeting all the aforementioned needs requires research, particularly in the area of behavioral change, including examination of the effects of the measurements themselves. The two most common measures, dietary recall and observation of school plate waste, are both subject to major errors. In addition, a theoretical framework for nutrition education and evaluation must be developed; building such a framework requires better communications among researchers. Finally, administrators and policymakers must be educated about realistic expectations for nutrition program evaluation.

Teacher Training.   Teacher training in nutrition education is subject to the same problems as other forms of nutrition education. Research observations in the field are often limited to changes in teacher knowledge or amounts of training completed rather than training outcomes—that is, whether the nutrition education programs conducted for students are effective, or whether they are conducted at all. Objectives, measures, and instrumentation are needed to design and evaluate teacher training programs. Little is known about teacher attitudes: what attitudes contribute to effective nutrition education, and how can training programs foster such attitudes? Teacher behaviors and student program outcomes are also in need of research. We do know that in both cases knowledge alone is not sufficient to produce appropriate behaviors, and we are not even sure what the appropriate behaviors are. Finally, in addition to training, teachers need suitable materials and curricula and the support of parents and school administrators.

Food Service Personnel.   NET legislation and regulations provide for training for food service personnel in all areas, not only nutrition education, in the interest of maximizing the benefits of school feeding programs by producing meals that are cheaper, nutritionally superior, and more acceptable to potential program participants.

Many aspects of the training of food service personnel are more readily determined and evaluated than are most aspects of nutrition education. Food preparation, lunchroom management, and even nutrition-related behaviors are readily measured, for the desired behavior is known, meal patterns are defined, and measures of cost-effectiveness exist. The training of food service personnel has a relatively long history dating back to the establishment of the school lunch program in the 1940s. Of course, school food services have extensive experience with actual food and food handling, enabling the school food service personnel to make a major contribution to the "hands-on" aspects of child nutrition education.

Nutrition education training is desired by a large number of personnel at all skill levels, although there is little evidence to suggest that training would help food service personnel contribute to nutrition education for students. Teachers and administrators have historically not been included in food service training, but within the last few years, and especially under the NET program, joint training has been increasing.

Nutrition Education for Preschoolers.   For the very young child, knowledge and behavior are closely linked. Nutrition education for this age group is of necessity experiential rather than didactic, and a wealth of curricula and activity guidelines is available. Unfortunately, much of the food-related activity now conducted with young children is strongly oriented toward skills other than nutritional ones: food preparation activities may be well-planned, but they produce sweets or other foods that lack nutritive value. Teachers' awareness of good nutrition principles and familiarity with suitable activities enables them to conduct appropriate nutrition education activities. Much of the research related to nutrition experiences for children focuses on known problem areas, particularly a child's reluctance to eat fruits and vegetables or to try new foods. Unfortunately, behavior modification techniques, which seem effective, have used sweets as reinforcers. Appropriate research designs are needed.

Elementary School Children.   Nutrition education for elementary school children is no exception to the pervading emphasis on cognitive change. Most curricula emphasize cognitive achievement, often at a low level of sophistication. Recent curricula are more likely to include behavioral objectives, but they do not always provide the teacher with evaluation materials or methods. The main reason for this is the lack of definitions of desirable behaviors and the instrumentation with which to assess them. Many curricula focus on outdated nutrition concerns rather than current issues, such as obesity and fat, salt, sugar, and fiber consumption. Most are based on input from nutrition professionals but do not draw on the expertise of psychologists, media experts, sociologists, and others concerned with the large picture of nutrition behavior. Some locally produced innovative curricula have addressed these programmatic needs in terms of local students' needs and concerns, apparently with good results, but these efforts are not well communicated. Also, little is known about the special program needs of minority, low-income, or bilingual students.

The available literature reports on only a fraction of the work actually being done. Although a literature search revealed only thirteen studies which reported objective assessments of nutrition education programs for this age group, eleven studies found increases in nutrition knowledge, as defined and measured by each study. Eleven studies used behavioral measures to assess outcomes, but only four found any improvements. This result may be due not to lack of behavioral impacts, but to the weak methodologies used to measure behavioral change or to the short time frames involved.

Secondary School Children.   Adolescents are in a developmental phase that presents unique opportunities and difficulties for nutrition education. Undergoing great physical, psychological, and emotional changes, adolescents experiment with behaviors and are amenable to outside influences, although peers are the preferred models. Concern with body image, weight, hair, and skin can be used as a starting point for health education, particularly nutrition, as can social and environmental concerns. The problems of this group are numerous: nutritional deficiencies, overweight and underweight, pregnancy, and athletics all are common enough to indicate that students need to be better equipped to make sound nutrition choices.

Again, a literature search uncovered few reported studies (ten in this case) suggesting that we need to develop an information base for program design and evaluation, as well as better systems of communication. Current work is hampered by lack of funds, time, and appropriate methodologies. Many curricula and programs fail to treat students' perceived needs and concerns as legitimate. They also overlook social influences on attitudes and behavior; do not coordinate efforts by parents, administrators, and food service personnel; and fail to help students take responsibility for their own health and diet.

Conclusions

Clearly, the nutrition education field has many shortcomings. All of these shortcomings can ultimately be addressed, but a greater degree of coordination will be required. This volume and its sponsorship by a federal agency suggest that the needed coordination may be forthcoming.

BIBLIOGRAPHY

Ferb, T. E. et al. 1980. *The Nutrition Education and Training Program: A Status Report 1977–1980,* Volume I. Cambridge, Mass.: Abt Associates Inc.

Whitehead, F. E. 1973. Nutrition Education Research. *World Review of Nutrition and Diet.* 17: 91–149.

1

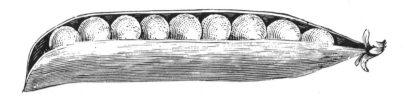

A CONCEPTUAL FRAMEWORK FOR INDIVIDUAL NUTRITION

Joanne P. Nestor

INTRODUCTION

To compare and evaluate nutrition education studies and programs, we must have a basis for comparison—a conceptual framework for the complex interrelationships among the many factors that determine an individual's nutritional status. Since our search of the literature detected no comprehensive framework, we present a new model in this chapter (see Figure 1). Based upon a model developed by the author and staff at Abt Associates Inc. (Abt Associates Inc. 1979), it does not attempt to suggest causal relationships (the state of the research does not permit such inferences), nor does it show all the possible interrelationships among the factors shown. For example, a significant relationship may exist between the private sector (a secondary influence) and biological food needs (a primary influence): the more television a child watches, the less time he spends exercising, reducing his caloric needs. Although such a relationship seems probable, to our knowledge it has not been formally documented. What this model can do is suggest the larger picture of which nutrition education is a part and provide a basis for discussion of the relationships among these factors. In the following discussion we define the factors used in the model and illustrate some of the known and possible relationships among these factors. Because the chapters that follow examine school-based nutrition education, we focus in this chapter on the factors closely related to school activities.

SECONDARY INFLUENCES

A child's *family*—parents, siblings, and other household members—influences the child's nutritional status by providing much of his food, particularly during the early years, and by setting an example for the child in food selection and consumption. The family establishes the patterns for many of the child's feeding activities and can also influence eating patterns through the degree of flexibility allowed the child in developing his own food preferences. Of course, the parents have also provided the child with the genetic basis for his food needs.

Although the influence of the family decreases as the child grows older and more independent, it is a major influence during

Figure 1
Individual Nutrition Influences, Responses, and Impacts

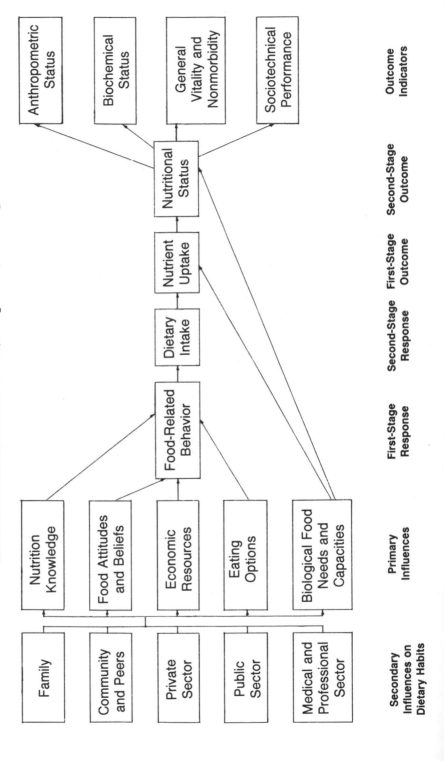

the early years.* Parental involvement is an important aspect of nutrition education programs, both in and out of school, because the parents' actions and words can markedly enhance or hinder educational efforts.

The *community and peers* influence a child's intake through expressed or implied attitudes toward specific foods. Cultural beliefs and activities can affect intake, particularly ceremonies, holidays, and other traditional events associated with consumption of or abstention from certain foods. Community programs frequently provide nutrition education or meals for children. The influence of peers, both in and out of school, increases as the child reaches adolescence.

The *private sector* affects food choices and availability through a number of competitive mechanisms. The food industry supplies an ever-increasing variety of convenience foods, from "TV dinners" to premixed beverages and prepared cereals to ready-to-eat desserts and snack foods, and fast food restaurants offer an easy meal option. Moreover, radio, television, magazines, billboards, and newspapers remind us of the abundance of convenience foods. Food giveaways provide consumption experiences which the providers hope the recipients will seek to repeat.

The private sector also is primarily responsible for the quantity and quality of food available to the consumer. The quantity of food an individual consumes has (theoretically, at least) an upper limit, unlike his capacity for most other consumer goods, and the variety of unprocessed foods in this system leaves little potential for additions. Therefore, growth for much of the food industry relies upon increasing one's share of a relatively inflexible market, resulting in competition among novel products—in this case, processed foods. Competition between unprocessed and processed foods is limited, because the latter are usually more profitable. As children's purchasing power and their independence in making food choices increase, so does their potential as consumers of profitable foods.

Many food and vitamin producers or associations contribute to nutrition education by producing educational materials or curricula. Among the most active are the National Dairy Council and the Dairy Council Inc. (originally of California), which produce

---

*The major influences of parents on young children are discussed in Chapter Five.

popular curricula discussed in the following chapters. Industry materials frequently focus on a particular food, nutrient, or belief, and some are not suitable for use without a broader program which can put their messages in perspective (Harty 1979).

The *public sector,* including public agencies at the local, state, and federal levels, influences consumption by increasing access to specific foods or to general sources of food and by educating the public. In-kind programs, such as School Lunch, Breakfast, Special Milk, and the Special Supplemental Food Program for Women, Infants, and Children (WIC), influence eating habits by providing foods and offering particular food choices. The Food Stamp Program increases access to food without restricting choices. Direct aid, such as welfare, provides increased discretionary income, which may be used for food purchases. Indirectly, state and other government agencies provide consultation, assistance, and facilities, which may help to increase or improve the food supply. Emergency aid programs, such as disaster relief, help maintain access to foods.

As the major funding source of the Nutrition Education and Training (NET) Program, the federal government is enabling local schools and school districts to provide students, teachers, and food service personnel with the ability to improve their nutritional status and their impact on the nutritional status of the community. Within the school system, inputs to nutrition education programs can be detailed, as in Gillespie's model (Gillespie 1979) of the family and school environments (see Figure 2).

The *medical and professional sector* serves nutrition by conducting research in agriculture, behavior, and dietetics and by providing nutrition counseling to programs and individuals. Most nutrition education activities conducted by medical personnel are directed toward individuals with existing nutrition-related health problems, as contrasted with the preventive and group orientations of school-based programs. Dietitians and community nutritionists work with groups on a preventive basis, including consultation with teachers and school programs. In view of teachers' dearth of nutrition expertise (see Chapter Three), this resource should be utilized more actively.

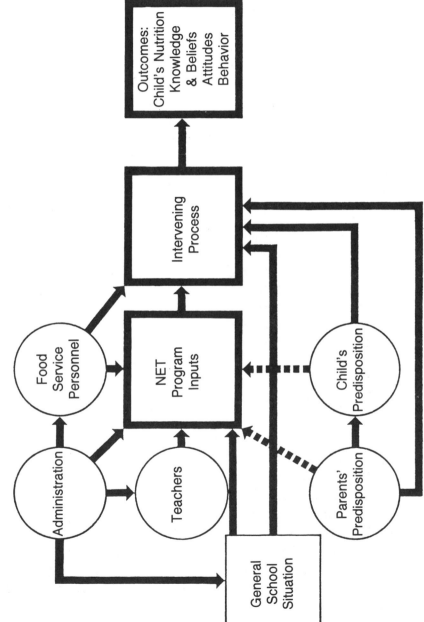

Figure 2
Gillespie's Model for Evaluation of the Nutrition Education and
Training (NET) Program.

PRIMARY INFLUENCES

Improving *nutrition knowledge,* the cognitive aspect of an individual's nutrition framework, is a goal of many nutrition education efforts conducted by the persons and organizations constituting the secondary influences. We must examine the outcomes of these efforts to identify the features which distinguish the successful ones. Adequate knowledge is necessary for an individual to make food-related decisions, although knowledge alone is by no means sufficient. Since individuals have different nutritional needs and resources, the knowledge they need also varies; nutrition education programs must take these varying needs into account.

An additional factor for consideration is that individuals entering a nutrition education program already possess some nutrition information, which varies in amount and accuracy from one individual to another. In order to meet educational needs most effectively, programs need to know their students' starting points—the base upon which new information is attached—and the ways in which such information has been acquired. Olson and Sims (1980) describe several methods of measuring aspects of nutritional knowledge to describe the psychological processes involved in acquiring nutrition information, storing it in memory, retrieving it at a later time, and using it in decision making. They present a research strategy based on the concept of information processing. Further research may reveal how different types of knowledge structures are related to the use of new nutrition information in making correct food choices. For example, a person who has not yet learned the meaning of "nutrient" will not comprehend information about a specific nutrient, such as Vitamin C. Additional research is also needed to identify the knowledge required to make sound decisions in today's complex food system. Many programs are based on food groupings or key nutrients, which may not be relevant to current concerns with excessive salt, fats, and calories rather than deficient nutrients.

Attitude, or affect, refers to an individual's feelings toward and evaluation of some object, person, issue, or event. Attitudes are most commonly measured on a bipolar scale indicating favorableness or unfavorableness toward the topic in question. *Beliefs* link objects to attributes, or link two facts (cognitive), and have the attribute of strength—the perceived likelihood that the object has (or is associated with) the attribute in question (Fishbein and Ajzen 1975). For example, an individual's attitude toward potato chips may be that he likes them (more or less intently), whereas his belief may be that potato chips (the object) are bad for a person (the attribute); yet that belief may not be as strong as his belief that food additives are bad for a person.

Beliefs, like knowledge, may be more or less accurate in terms of dietetic information; attitudes may be more or less appropriate in their relationship to desirable nutrition behavior. Although beliefs and attitudes are no doubt interrelated as are items of nutrition knowledge, no system for assessing and relating them has been proposed, although Olson and Sims's (1980) knowledge structure depends to some extent on beliefs about the facts reported.

Among the strongest beliefs are those that relate foods to preventive or curative roles in determining health status. Other powerful sociocultural beliefs or attitudes include religious prohibitions of certain foods and children's dislike of foods that are not aesthetically acceptable to them.

The Interagency Committee on Nutrition Education (1972) cited extensive evidence and professional opinion that lack of motivation (that is, a negative attitude toward the importance of nutrition) is the major obstacle to improving the nutrition behavior of the public. Public interest in nutrition issues has grown since the early 1970s, as evidenced by increasing press coverage, book sales, course attendance, and the like, but student attitudes toward the importance and relevance of nutrition remain an obstacle.

Economic resources can bias or limit intake. Total family income and the proportion spent for food affect access to food and attitudes toward it, as do supplementary resources, such as food stamps. Variations in diets can also be caused by seasonal availability and price fluctuations of produce which is not available or affordable year round. Children's allowances and other spending money are often utilized to increase access to foods not available through other sources, such as home and school meals.

Although economic resources may be the limiting factor governing access to food in the United States, food supply factors not included in this model may have significant effects on access to food under other circumstances. Transportation, social status within the family or a larger social group, and availability of quantitatively and qualitatively adequate fuel and water supplies are rarely significant factors in the United States but may be overriding concerns in countries with different agricultural and socioeconomic constraints.

Because the U.S. food supply is more than adequate and because most families can afford adequate diets, the determining factor in dietary adequacy in the United States is often the appropriateness of the choices that are made among *eating options*. The issue of choice is the focus of most nutrition education programs. Under conditions of increasing food prices and general economic distress, individuals seeking to economize on food may adjust their eating habits in positive ways, by cutting back on "empty calories," "junk foods," excessive calories, or meat intake, or negatively, by cutting back on foods essential to the quality of the diet. At such times, consumer education in nutrition can help maintain or even improve diet quality.

Children are presented with a variety of eating options. In addition to food provided at home (or through the home, such as picnics or lunches for school), breakfast, lunch, extra milk, or some combination of these are offered to students in school. Many schools also have vending machines or allow students to visit neighborhood stores and restaurants during school hours. Outside of school, children with financial resources can choose from a wide array of food sources: restaurants, snack bars, ice cream parlors, soda fountains, vending machines, street vendors, corner grocers, delicatessens, specialty food shops, convenience stores, and supermarkets. Children without financial resources are frequently given food by friends and neighbors.

A popular nutrition education tool is the "tasting party," which provides opportunities (and encouragement) to try unfamiliar foods. The educational effects of exposure to foods and regular access to them should be examined systematically. Such activities often resemble behavior modification exercises and take advantage of peer pressure or modeling to enhance their impact.

The child's *biological food needs and capacities* are determined both genetically and environmentally. Although genetic makeup determines an individual's optimum potential, it can be limited by environment, and the supply of nutrients is believed to have more effect on growth than any other environmental factor. Nutrition involves the food supply and the whole chain of body processes that draw upon nutritional intake to support the growth, maintenance, and repair of tissues. The absolute biological need for food is hunger; appetite, which is the feeling of a need for food, can be evoked by time, the presence of food, social conditioners, or other food cues. Biological food needs for calories and other nutrients are determined by an individual's age, sex, size, health, and level of activity. In a perfectly tuned body the appetite regulates food intake, which supplies a suitable balance of food energy and other nutrients for the activities performed. But for children exposed to many eating opportunities, food cues are frequent, and the appetite may override the balance mechanism, resulting in inappropriate intake. Education can help the child distinguish physical need for foods from other factors influencing food choices. Nutrition programs must recognize the special needs of students who are undernourished, pregnant, obese, participating in athletics, and so forth.

RESPONSES

Influenced by the environmental factors described above, the individual decides whether to take advantage of a particular eating opportunity and, if so, what and how much to eat. The outcome of this decision is the individual's *food-related behavior,* which determines nutritional intake. Most nutrition education research that includes behavioral observations examines the effects of varying one or two of the primary influences. Little is known about the interactions among the influences or the ways in which, as a group, they interact within the individual's decision-making process. A better understanding of this process would make nutrition education programs more effective, but, as Chapter Two on evaluation will show, such research is difficult to conduct given our current understanding of the primary influences.

The foods actually consumed represent the individual's *dietary intake,* which the body depends upon for the nutrients it requires. Regardless of the individual's perceptions, the body's requirements can be expressed in terms of nutrients; the amounts needed depend upon the individual's needs for growth, maintenance, and repair and on the efficiency with which nutrients are drawn from the foods ingested. The adequacy of dietary intake is frequently used as a basis for judging the appropriateness of an individual's food behavior. However, this criterion has several disadvantages. First, without extensive metabolic assessments, one does not know an individual's nutrient requirements. The National Academy of Science's Recommended Daily Allowances (RDAs) are statistically adequate for 97.5 percent of the population for each nutrient; therefore, 2.5 percent of the population may consume the RDA of a nutrient and still have an inadequate intake, while 97.5 percent of the population may consume less than the RDA and not be at risk. Therefore, dietary inadequacy and functional nutritional deficiency are not the same thing. Second, even determining what nutrients an individual has consumed is difficult: reported and observed intakes are not reliable or adequate indicators, and food composition varies according to source and preparation. Third, RDAs have not yet been established for all nutrients known to be essential. Frequently, "major" or "key" nutrients have been used as indicators of dietary adequacy, but these are the very nutrients now used to enrich or fortify many highly refined foods—notably breakfast cereals—which are lacking in most other nutrients and thus are not reliable indicators (Huenemann 1971).

RELATIONSHIPS AMONG KNOWLEDGE, BELIEFS, ATTITUDES, AND BEHAVIOR

Although this review does not focus on the interrelationships among the factors modeled, one set of relationships must be addressed. Many people assume that an increase in knowledge will produce a change in attitude, which in turn will result in improved behavior. This assumption underlies most knowledge-oriented nutrition programs, but we have no conclusive evidence that it is correct. Indeed, the prevalence of obesity, in spite of common knowledge that obesity is caused by overeating, is abundant evidence to the contrary. Weight loss clinics, books, and fad diets thrive, and many individuals manage to lose weight. But even those who do lose weight often regain it. Clearly, the relationships among knowledge, beliefs, attitudes, and behavior are complex and not simply a causal chain.

The roots of this assumption of causality lie in consistency theory, which includes the psychological concept of cognitive dissonance. Many educators assume that if an individual acquires knowledge or beliefs that are inconsistent with his behavior, the need to resolve this dissonance will cause him to adjust his attitudes and behavior appropriately in order to relieve the ensuing psychic distress. Or will it? Smokers know about lung cancer; most obese persons believe that overweight is undesirable and that it is caused by overeating.

Contento (1979) notes that Piagetian learning theory maintains that when newly acquired knowledge contradicts that which is already assimilated, a state of "disequilibrium" is created, forcing "accommodation" through the reorganization of existing reasoning strategies. At the points of disequilibrium, persons are receptive to suggestions that might assist them in resolving the contradictions they are experiencing. Contento found that graduate-level nutrition students did not always use the type of formal reasoning that consistency theory assumes is used in adapting to new knowledge. She proposed a learning process designed to encourage the use of formal reasoning. Since children of school age also have not reached this level of causal reasoning, we cannot assume that they will utilize infusions of nutrition knowledge as consistency theory would dictate.

Editorializing as president of the Society for Nutrition Education, Guthrie observed that although "primarily we [the Society for Nutrition Education] are committed to programs which increase the amount of information which people have about sound nutrition practices ..." "... many who are well-informed retain very faulty dietary habits" (1978, p. 57). Indeed, many persons who have severe problems with weight, drugs, alcohol, and so forth are among the best-informed, but for many others a little knowledge about the risks involved seems to have been adequate to produce the behavior desired by the educators. As Olson and Sims state, "behavior such as food choice can be seen as a function of the cognitive processes and states [among which they include beliefs and attitudes] that intervene between exposure to a nutrition education message and the actual selecting of foods" (1980, p.158). Guthrie concludes that "the challenge for us who practice nutrition education is to find ways in addition to providing information to change the nutrition-related behavior of those who are not acting on the information they have" (1978, p. 57). (As previous sections of this discussion have indicated, nutrition education programs in the United States can reasonably assume that most individuals have physical and economic access to a nutritionally adequate food supply.) Margaret Mead, however, has contended that the first question we must ask is not "How do we change food habits?" but rather "How do food habits change?"

The Agricultural Extension Service of the U.S. Department of Agriculture produced a model of acceptance of change (Swanson 1972) that uses the following sequence:

1. awareness,
2. interest,
3. evaluation,
4. trial,
5. adoption.

Hochbaum and Rosenstock (Swanson 1972) proposed that an individual, before taking a health-related action, must:

1. perceive the issue as important,
2. believe himself to be susceptible to the condition,
3. believe the problem is serious,
4. not perceive the intensity of the threat with such great anxiety as to paralyze his ability to act, and
5. believe the action to be effective and be able to take it.

The problem of motivation, discussed above in regard to attitudes, also arises here in "interest" and the first three of Hochbaum's items. This aspect of nutrition education has been neglected. Not only do many students exhibit apathy or hostility toward nutrition per se, they are often not motivated to learn the concepts presented. The relevance of program content should be examined in relation to students' concerns or to the potential for increasing student interest (Kirk, Hamrick, and McAfee 1975). Although these models seem to assume the progression from knowledge to behavior, they also suggest some of the obstacles to behavioral change perceived by Olson and Sims (1980). Most knowledge-oriented nutrition education programs focus on dietetic facts rather than information or other strategies directed at developing the interest, evaluation, and trial phases proposed by the Extension Service, nor do they address development of beliefs and attitudes, which Hochbaum contends is essential. If these processes must occur in order for appropriate nutrition behavior to be induced, then nutrition educators must consider them to design effective programs. Subsequent chapters will report on the findings of a few studies assessing behavioral changes induced by knowledge-oriented programs, but on the whole research into the relationships among these elements is lacking.

Swanson suggests that even our assumption regarding the *ordering* of changes in knowledge, attitudes, and behavior may not always be correct. Behavior may change before attitudes, and attitudes are more resistant to change than was previously supposed (Swanson 1972). Chapter Five, reviewing preschool nutrition education, cites several programs that use behavior modification techniques and do result in increased consumption of certain foods, presumably reflecting the children's more positive attitudes toward these foods. Swanson notes that alternative responses to cognitive dissonance, other than modification of attitude to suit behavior, are rationalization, denial, and differentiation, all of which are observed among individuals with persistent health-related behavioral problems (such as smoking).

Nutrition education must address psychosocial factors as well as dietetic data, and, as Guthrie notes, we should not be any less scientific about the former than we are about the latter: "We should not cling to any method of education unless we have evidence that it brings about desirable habits of food consumption" (Guthrie 1978, p. 58). Chapter Two examines the status of evaluation techniques.

OUTCOMES

Nutrient uptake from foods consumed is achieved through the processes of digestion, metabolism, and absorption. Individual variations play a major role in these processes. Nutritional need can also influence uptake; for instance, iron is absorbed less efficiently if body stores are adequate. Nutrient uptake may be impeded by the presence of intestinal parasites.

Nutritional status has been defined as the condition of an individual's health as influenced by intake and utilization of nutrients. Nutritional status is determined by correlating information obtained from physical and biochemical studies.

OUTCOME INDICATORS

Anthropometric status reveals short- and long-term adequacy of intake. Stature (height), besides reflecting genetic potential, also depends upon the intake of calories, protein, calcium, and other nutrients during periods of growth. Characteristics of skeletal development can indicate nutritional inadequacies in an individual's past. Weight responds more rapidly to variations in nutritional intake, primarily caloric intake. Skin folds can be examined on various parts of the body to measure thickness of subcutaneous fat, a more accurate indicator of adiposity than weight alone. Other measures can also be used in gauging growth and maturity.

Weight is one of the few readily observed and readily influenced measures of nutritional status. Obesity is a major health and nutritional problem, and one with which the public is actively concerned, although often ineffectively.

Biochemical status can reveal variations in short-term intake and need for changes in nutrient intake. Because most measures of biochemical status are laboratory procedures involving assessment of blood, urine, and other bodily tissues or fluids, they are not practical evaluation measures for most programs. Nevertheless, they do constitute a valuable indicator of nutritional status of individuals and groups and have been used in some of the research discussed in subsequent chapters.

The adequacy of an individual's intake influences his *general vitality and nonmorbidity.* Well-nourished and well-developed organisms have a greater resistance to infection; are more vigorous, more efficient, and live longer; and are characterized by superior posture, musculature, coloring, dentition, and digestive ability. Although the mutually reinforcing relationship between infection and overt malnutrition is well-established (Scrimshaw, Taylor, and Gordon 1968), less is known about interactions between disease and borderline nutritional intake. Vitamin deficiency diseases are now uncommon in the United States, but iron deficiency anemia is common, as are nutrition-related diseases of the circulatory system. Indeed, nutrition-related degenerative diseases are now among the most common causes of death. Medicine may be able to prevent infectious diseases and assuage the effects of poor diets, but individuals can rely only upon themselves to make the everyday dietary decisions that can preserve their health.

The individual's *sociotechnical performance* is affected by nutritional status. The well–nourished individual exhibits more buoyant energy, vigor, and interest, as well as prompt and adequate recovery from fatigue. The body functions well: appetite and digestion are good, the nervous system is stable, endurance is good, and sleep is sound and refreshing. The Iowa Breakfast Studies addressed the measurement of the physical and mental effects of meals, but few if any current nutrition education programs attempt to do so. Many school breakfast programs report that school attendance, performance, and discipline have improved (U.S. General Accounting Office 1980).

BIBLIOGRAPHY

Abt Associates Inc. 1979. The Evaluation of the Impact of the National School Lunch and Breakfast Programs. RFP no. 25–FNS–79. Cambridge, Mass.: Abt Associates Inc. (August 21).

Contento, Isobel. 1979. Measuring and Enhancing Reasoning Abilities of Nutrition Graduate Students—A Piagetian Approach. *J. Nutr. Educ.* 11:184.

Fishbein, M., and Ajzen, I. 1975. Belief, Attitude, Intention and Behavior: An Introduction to Theory and Research. Reading, Mass.: Addison-Wesley Publishing Co.

Gillespie, A. 1979. A Framework for Evaluation of the Nutrition Education and Training Program. Paper presented at the Twelfth Annual Meeting of the Society for Nutrition Education, 22–25 July 1979, San Francisco, Calif.

Guthrie, H.A. 1978. Is Education Not Enough? *J. Nutr. Educ.* 10:57.

Harty, S. 1979. Hucksters in the Classroom. Washington, D.C.: Center for the Study of Resonsive Law.

Huenemann, R.L. 1971. A Review of Teenage Nutrition in the United States. In *Proceedings of National Nutrition Education Conference.* Washington, D.C.: U.S. Department of Agriculture. Pub. No. 1254:37.

Interagency Committee on Nutrition Education. 1972. Nutrition Education for Youth. *J. Home Econ.* 64:34.

Kirk, R.H.; Hamrick, M.; and McAfee, D.C. 1975. Nutrition in Health Instruction: The Tennessee Health Education Project. *J. Nutr. Educ.* 7:68.

Olson, J.C., and Sims, L.S.. 1980. Assessing Nutrition Knowledge from an Information Processing Perspective. *J. Nutr. Educ.* 12:157.

Scrimshaw, N.S.; Taylor, C.E.; and Gordon, J.E. 1968. Interactions of Nutrition and Infection. Geneva: World Health Organization.

Swanson, J.C. 1972. Second Thoughts on Knowledge and Attitude Effects upon Behavior. *J. Sch. Health* 42:363.

U.S. General Accounting Office. 1980. Major Factors Inhibit Expansion of the School Breakfast Program. Draft of proposed report. Washington, D.C.: U.S. General Accounting Office.

2

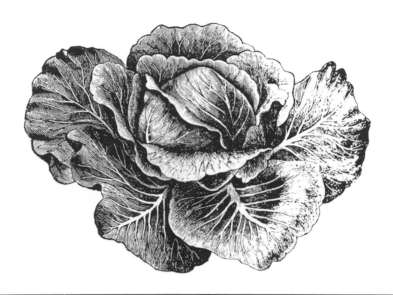

EVALUATION OF
NUTRITION
EDUCATION:
A REVIEW

Judy K. Brun

INTRODUCTION

Today, most nutrition education programs include an expanded evaluation component in order to provide evidence of the program's value and effectiveness and to guide decision making. In describing the need for evaluation of nutrition education programs, Guthrie states: "We would not promote a class of foods without evidence of its contribution to good nutrition, and we should not cling to any method of [nutrition] education unless we have evidence that it brings about desirable habits in food consumption" (1978, p. 58).

Attention in the literature to the kind of evaluation conducted before the 1940s is limited. However, references in recent writings to earlier work give some indication of its focus. Whitehead notes that early program successes were measured in terms of ". . . defects corrected, gains in weight, and physical improvement" (1957, p. 883) and that many early programs focused on the underweight child (1973). Changes in height, weight, skin fold, blood chemistry, and other anthropometric indicators were emphasized. There was little attention to increased knowledge gain and changes in food habits. However, the nutrition education work done by Mary Swartz Rose in the 1920s emphasized formative evaluation, because it was conducted to help clarify nutritional concepts through improved units of study (Todhunter 1965).

McKenzie and Mumford (1965) reviewed studies conducted in the 1940s and 1950s of changes in food habits as related to education. For example, they cited Lewin's classic 1943 study comparing two educational techniques for increasing consumption of heart, brain, and kidney. They criticized many studies for their failure to make objective assessments, insufficient consideration of long-term change, and inadequate control groups and suggested that the purely technical devices for gathering evaluation data had to be improved.

Improvements in the evaluation of nutrition education programs have gone hand in hand with improvements in nutrition education itself and with the increased emphasis on accountability that has permeated education since the mid-1960s. At that time the federal government, which was providing increased funds for educational programs, insisted upon evaluation of these programs to show that taxpayer funds were being spent wisely. Educators around the country became more involved in evaluation, the theoretical base became more sophisticated, and methodology and techniques improved.

In the following review of evaluation in nutrition education, methodology and procedures for gathering data will be outlined. Major attention will be given to needs assessment as a first step in setting direction for program development, formative evaluation to guide revisions during development of programs or curricula, and the effectiveness of programs or curricula that have been implemented.

THE PURPOSE OF EVALUATION

Most models of evaluation call for a clear statement of program goals as a first step in designing the evaluation study. These goal or outcome statements establish the purpose for the study and suggest the program components that will be evaluated.

Statements about the purpose of evaluating nutrition education often reflect professional positions or philosophical views. For example, Congressman Frederick Richmond, in describing the goal of the Congress in nutrition education evaluation, makes the following statement:

The agencies of the Federal Government . . . need to be able to justify their programs on the basis of logic, research and feedback. The old numbers game of counting prints that leave the shelves, and faces encountered in meeting rooms is pointless. If the Congress is to provide the dollars and the policy initiatives to fuel a national nutrition education program, we must be assured that it will accomplish significant improvement in the health and well-being of citizens. (1977, p. 151)

Audrey Maretzki, former director of the Food and Nutrition Service, U.S. Department of Agriculture, sees a broader focus for the evaluation of nutrition education. In referring to the nationwide evaluation of the federally funded Nutrition Education and Training Program, she comments, "Information derived from this study undoubtedly will affect the future of nutrition education in the United States. Since the role of research and evaluation in nutrition education has only begun to be recognized, we can expect that whatever we learn will advance the state of this fledgling art"

(Maretzki 1979b, p. 176). In this sense, evaluation could be viewed as a formative study describing the effectiveness of a model nutrition education program as it is being developed and implemented. However, Maretzki states that the real test will not be in the numbers of teachers trained, curricular materials developed, parents reached, or children taught, nor only in terms of health, but in ". . . whether the children of the 1980s will themselves enjoy the benefits of optimal nutrition and ultimately be able to bring nutrition ideas to bear on the range of social, economic and political problems which involve decision-making about food" (1979b, p. 180).

The American Dietetic Association, in its 1973, 1974, and 1978 policy statements on nutrition education, places emphasis on nutrition specifics in describing evaluation needs. These statements stress the assessment of nutritional needs as part of the evaluation component guiding the development of nutrition education programs. The 1978 statement specifies:

> Evaluation must be part of all nutritional endeavors, with measurable objectives constructed to determine the effectiveness of the programs. Depending on resources, facilities and methods of evaluation will vary. Appropriate stated measurements of indicators may be: increased nutrition knowledge; changes in food purchasing and selection; behavior and actual health outcomes as reflected in objective physical measurements or biochemical data. Resources should be allocated for meaningful and objective data collection and analysis so that the program can be restructured as necessary to achieve stated goals. (American Dietetic Association 1978, p. 305)

The statement seems to imply that a major deterrent to effective evaluation is lack of measurable objectives, that once these are "appropriate" and "stated" the evaluation can proceed with little problem, and that the primary purpose is to provide information for program revision. There is also the erroneous implication that the methods of evaluation depend largely on resources available to the evaluator.

Concern about the purpose of evaluation also comes from the academic sector. For example, as McCool observes:

> Evaluation studies can be ineffective if: (a) They are not planned to support program decision-making; (b) The timing, format, and precision are not geared to user needs; (c) The

results are inadequately communicated to decision-makers;
(d) The studies are addressed to unanswerable questions and
produce inconclusive results. (1979, p. 564)

Ramsey and Cloyd's (1979) experience illustrates the tensions that
result when program evaluations are expected to show unrealistic
results. They conducted an evaluation of the Expanded Food and
Nutrition Education Programs in the state of Minnesota. In addition to evaluating objectives directly related to nutrition, they were
asked to look at other diverse objectives written to "enrich" the
program and increase the appeal for funding, such as decreased
feelings of powerlessness, greater civic participation, and greater
reliance on professionals for help in solving problems. They found
it difficult to provide hard data for these objectives and suggest the
need to distinguish between those objectives that can demonstrably
be achieved and those that cannot.

Several other controversies affect the purpose of evaluation in
nutrition education. The issue of rigor versus significance in designing an evaluation study is raised by Green (1977). If evaluation
results are to be generalizable to a variety of situations, educational treatments and procedures must be rigorously defined. Rigorous
evaluations may provide new research knowledge but not the information needed to decide how best to implement educational programs under varying conditions.

Another issue is that of effectiveness versus economy of scale.
Funds are often not available to study nutrition education programs on a nationwide basis without evaluating programs as they
affect a cross-section of the nation's population; there is only limited information with which to determine program effectiveness for
various groups of people.

Long- versus short-term evaluation continues to be a problem,
too. Longitudinal studies are desirable because change in behavior
occurs slowly. However, the difficulties of conducting longitudinal
studies in nutrition education, as in other fields, are many.

As technology develops, it is possible to change the criteria for
designing evaluation studies and analyzing data. With the development of new statistical programs and computer facilities, evaluation can become more sophisticated. For example, at the present
time, the adequacy of foods consumed is determined primarily on
the basis of short-term, self-report data, using the criteria of food

groups and major nutrients. Home computers and programs using more sophisticated nutritional criteria may produce more accurate information about what people actually purchase, prepare, and eat over long periods of time.

The objectives of evaluation studies reported in the nutrition education literature are not always stated. The reason may be lack of consensus about the desired outcomes of nutrition education programs, lack of knowledge about educational evaluation, or a belief that the objectives are implied. When objectives are not clearly outlined, however, it makes an evaluation of the evaluation itself very difficult, because the criteria for judging the study are hard to establish. In this sense, the evaluation may lose credibility.

NEEDS, OBSTACLES, AND GOALS IN THE EVALUATION OF NUTRITION EDUCATION

Needs Assessment

Needs assessments, conducted to guide the development of programs, are essential to the success of nutrition education. Needs assessment can be used as a technique to enhance the effectiveness of nutrition education by improving the design of the program and by motivating the participants.

A major question related to the conduct of needs assessments is that of focus. In many cases, eventual participants, for example, a group of school age children, will be given tests to determine their current knowledge of nutrition. The total program is then based on this "needs assessment." Many activities related to the use of PL 95–166 funds seem to be of this nature. Ullrich suggests a broader focus for needs assessments, including:

> . . . public health figures on children's physical growth and school absence due to illness; number of children participating in school food service programs and their acceptance of these programs; types of training available to school food service workers and the number who participate; credential requirements and training in nutrition for teachers; number of teachers who have received any nutrition training; available

professional resources, including nutritionists, nutrition educators, and curriculum materials; and the kinds and sources of food and nutrition information existing outside the schools. (1978, p. 52)

Information about participants' knowledge and demographics are important to an effective needs assessment. However, as some of the following reviewed examples illustrate, other concerns also need to be included in a comprehensive needs assessment. A needs assessment should often include data about the nutritional status of the people who will receive the nutrition education program. A view gaining acceptance among nutrition educators is that the factors underlying and determining a target group's current food practices must be assessed in order to develop meaningful educational programs (Hochbaum 1977).

Numerous needs assessment studies can be found in the nutrition education literature. Several of these will be reviewed to illustrate the wide variety of approaches that can be taken and that need to be taken. Knowledge of these approaches can guide future work.

Family "readiness" refers to various sociological and nutritional dimensions of food habits existing within the family as a unit. Hertzler and Owen (1974) studied this concept in the belief that it offered a better strategy for nutrition education than information limited to level of knowledge. They considered the sociological matrix of a family an important needs assessment context in designing effective nutrition education programs.

Wishik and Van Der Vynckt used an unusual approach in their assessment of need. Instead of identifying those persons in the population who were most in need of nutrition education, they identified families among deprived populations ". . . in which a child between age six months and five years falls in the upper 25 percent in height and weight measurements" (1976, p. 38). They studied these families using anthropological techniques in examining sources of food, storage, preparation, and consumption to identify positive behavior that was culturally acceptable and could be used in developing nutrition education programs for other persons in the population who were not nutritionally positive. Although conducted on a Caribbean island and lacking specific guidelines for program design, this study could be used as a model for assessing needs in the United States.

Before developing school nutrition education programs, the National Dairy Council commissioned an outside group to conduct a needs assessment (Eash and Rasher 1976). With no assessment of students or parents, the focus was on teachers and administrators, who were asked about material and format preferences, various administrative problems that might interfere with the implementation of nutrition education programs, and the feasibility of implementing various programs within existing curricular structures. Although this is one kind of information approach that is useful in developing programs, it needs to be supplemented by other data.

Mapes (1977) used a classic curriculum development approach by surveying youths to determine their major nutritional concerns. She also questioned them about their preferred format for the delivery of nutrition education materials and, on this basis, designed comics focusing on three concepts.

Maretzki (1979a) conducted a similar but broader-scale study in Hawaii. Parents, teachers, and children were asked to list their various food activities. In the next step, parents and teachers compiled lists of seventeen nutrition education activities, ranked on scales of safety-danger and autonomy-control.

The importance of gathering data on current food practices is again illustrated in the work conducted by Terry, Bass, and Kolasa (1979). The researchers used anthropological approaches to gather information on the availability, safety, nutritive value, and the acceptability of foods among East Nicaraguan Miskito Indians. Such information was essential for planning and implementing nutrition education programs, especially in areas where the educators themselves were not familiar with relevant characteristics of the local population.

Yet another approach to needs assessment, prompted by scant information to guide state level programming and the use of PL 95–166 funds, was carried out by Levine, McChesney, and Brush (1979). They sent a questionnaire to all 205 high schools in New Jersey; received a 70 percent return; and gathered information about departments teaching nutrition, concepts taught, time allotted, types of methods and materials used, percent of students enrolled in courses in which nutrition education was taught, and background of the nutrition educator. These data were used to make suggestions about future programs.

Needs assessments conducted to guide nutrition education programming must be designed to meet the unique requirements of each situation. As the state of the art advances, more attention will be given to this evaluative step. Also, more creativity will be shown in the kinds of data gathered and the techniques used to gather it.

Obstacles

Many obstacles arise to inhibit the effective design and implementation of evaluation components, including formative, political, and economic difficulties.

The *lack of precise definitions* for critical terms used in data gathering and analysis often leads to unsophisticated evaluation designs and useless data (Guthrie 1977, Austin 1978). For example, there are no clear-cut definitions for the concepts of nutrition, nutritious food, or nutritious diet. The many variables involved (for example, sodium, cholesterol, and dietary deficiencies) even when identifiable, are often complicated or impossible to quantify. In another critical area, various attitudinal terms are not yet accurately or adequately defined (Foley, Hertzler, and Anderson 1979). This complicates the interpretation of many food habit studies because of the lack of necessary insight into food habit development and change.

The quality of evaluation of nutrition education cannot surpass that of the research knowledge available to guide these studies. More research in such areas as attitude formation and nutritional science can help provide a better understanding of the link between nutritional knowledge and food choice behaviors. This, in turn, can help nutrition educators more effectively develop objectives and teaching strategies for nutrition education programs and designs for evaluating program effectiveness.

A second obstacle is the *constraints imposed on and by teachers.* Although curriculum developers agree that evaluation procedures are an integral part of any curriculum or set of teaching plans, Cooper and Go found in their analysis of nutrition curriculum guides for elementary and secondary schools that: ". . . only 54 percent of guides included them. Forty-one percent included evaluative procedures on a frequent and consistent basis and 13 percent did so only occasionally. Only 23 percent frequently provided pretest procedures" (1976, p. 65). The missing evaluation component is a major problem. It is difficult and time-consuming for teachers to search for evaluation materials or to develop their own, but they face demands of accountability to students, administrators, and parents. They also recognize the need for evaluation of teaching and learning which leads to program improvement. Light (1978) echoed this concern by stating that one of the seven most frequently cited problems with existing national programs of nutrition education was the failure to include an evaluation component at any level.

Lack of cooperation on the part of teachers, food service personnel, or other program participants who feel threatened or annoyed by the evaluation process is another obstacle. Some do not appreciate the need for quantifiable or highly structured procedures and begrudge the imposition. Others believe that the evaluation could reveal inadequate performance on their part. Skeptics believe that evaluation results may be misinterpreted or otherwise abused in ways which reflect unfavorably on them, or which obviate the value of the project. Technical problems inherent in the development and administration of evaluation instruments can and do lead to such results, leaving participants unwilling to cooperate in further studies. As advances are made in instrumentation and in the appreciation of the role of human relations in evaluation, the impact of this obstacle will diminish.

Problems of methodology often affect the evaluation process. The methodologies and research settings used by social scientists and educators provide the theoretical base for research and evaluation in nutrition education more appropriately than do the methodologies of physical scientists. Variables are often difficult to identify and control, cooperation of subjects is often less than total, and conclusions and decisions often are reached after too little study.

Nevertheless, the fundamental question of how social determinants influence food selection patterns must be answered if a learner's food patterns are to be improved through an educational program. For example, Reaburn, Krondl, and Lau (1979) found that some of these social influences could be quantified and measured. They gave their subjects a food attitude questionnaire to describe food use frequency, availability, price, convenience, and prestige value of fifty-two food items. The researchers concluded that each food has its social profile, which varies among groups of people; once the job of developing these profiles for various groups is completed, better nutrition education strategies can be designed.

The evaluation process can be susceptible to *political considerations*. In the context of nutrition education, Austin states: "Some nutrition programs such as feeding are highly visible and, therefore, politically attractive. . . . The result is that nutritional impact becomes irrelevant as a program evaluation criterion" (1978, p. 2325). Yet political considerations in evaluation are not necessarily negative. The School Lunch Program is one example of a politically attractive program. Certain basic questions (such as "Why do it?") must be asked by those designing evaluation studies.

There appears to be little cross-referencing within the various studies and reports reviewed, especially among those papers concerned with evaluating the effectiveness of educational programs and materials. With few exceptions, the evaluators were not using each others' ideas, recommendations, or measurement instruments, but instead seemed to be "reinventing the wheel." This may indicate a lack of consensus about the goals of nutrition education programs, a misguided belief that it's not proper to use others' work, a reflection that evaluation of nutrition education is a new and developing area, or failure to conduct a thorough literature search. Just as researchers base their work on past developments, evaluators need to look to the literature for guidance in conducting future evaluation studies.

Financial constraints provide a dilemma for nutrition education evaluation. Although major attention is consistently given to the development and implementation of new programs and the administrative structures necessary for their function, evaluation components usually receive very small amounts of money. For example, in the mid-1970s the U.S. Office of Education, despite growing concern for evaluation, was spending less than .3 percent of total annual program appropriations on evaluation of federal education programs. When evaluation studies (which are often more expensive than research studies because of their depth and scope) are underfunded, they cannot be designed or conducted soundly or effectively.

Although many nutrition education programs are criticized for lack of adequate needs assessments before program development begins, the *lack of formative evaluation* during the development of nutrition education programs may be an even greater problem. In fact, few studies in the literature could truly be defined as formative evaluation. This dearth is unfortunate if the quality and the effectiveness of nutrition education are to improve, as Vivian Horner, Director of Research for "The Electric Company" at Children's Television Workshop, pointed out in her evaluation of the nutrition education television series "Mulligan Stew." Horner felt that the series lacked the minimal formative evaluation necessary to determine if student learning was indeed related to the intended purposes or outcomes of the program.

> If there is one thing we have learned at the Workshop, it is the importance of doing evaluative research prior to and during production, not simply after the fact, and of feeding the results back into the production process to insure the integration of educational intent with effective entertainment. If you don't insure this kind of research–production interaction, you must be very lucky indeed to end up with a product which is not an educational hodgepodge, however effective it may be in engaging the attention of its audience. Resultant learning is likely to be scant and uneven, where it might have been substantial and predictable. (Shapiro, Bale, and Scardino 1974, p.151).

The work of the National Dairy Council illustrates the use of formative evaluation in developing nutrition education curricula and programs. This organization contracts with an outside group to conduct evaluations of prototype materials during the developmental stages. For example, in the development of *FOOD . . . Your Choice* for grades kindergarten through six, the formative evaluation was conducted during an entire semester with prototype curriculum materials (Eash et al. 1977). The evaluation focused on student behavior, the learning environment of the classroom, and students' and teachers' reactions to the materials. Information from this piloting period was used to revise materials for final production. In 1979, during the development of *FOOD . . . Your Choice* for grades seven through ten, similar processes were used (Talmage and Rasher 1980). The outside evaluation group helped in learner verification of the first draft of the educational materials on an activity–by–activity basis in local classrooms. Based on this work, revised prototype materials were produced and tested at sites throughout the United States in the fall of 1979. Again, the focus in this testing was primarily on students' and teachers' reactions to the materials and on the learning environment, but also included looking at the materials as a complete package and initial work with student achievement. These extensive analyses of the activities and the overall curriculum package were used to make final revisions in the nutrition education materials.

Unfortunately, formative evaluation appears in other studies only when the materials are in final form. Due to the data gathered, the authors often summed up their studies with "because of the concerns identified in this research, further revisions of materials will be made."

The School Nutrition Education Curriculum Study at Pennsylvania State University has used formative evaluation techniques, but the procedures and results are not available. Others also have done work in this area, but their studies remain unpublished, perhaps because developers are hesitant to publicize identified problems or fail to recognize this factor as legitimate material for journal articles.

METHODOLOGIES

Guidelines for designing and conducting evaluation studies in nutrition education come from a variety of research and evaluation texts (for example, Campbell and Stanley 1973; Borg and Gall 1979; Bloom, Hastings, and Madaus 1971; Tuckman 1979). Our purpose is to review methodology as a guide to future evaluation developments, not to prepare a textbook.

Methodology and the related instrumentation involved in gathering data probably have more to do with the current state of the art than any of the dilemmas discussed in the preceeding section. However, interrelationships occur among the various aspects, for example, between politics and instruments, or finances and methods.

There are many aspects to the methodology of evaluation: cost effectiveness, evaluation of materials, quality of teacher preparation, and effectiveness of planning procedures. While these areas appear in specific studies reviewed in later sections, this section centers on three areas related to effectiveness in educating the students or clients of nutrition programs: (1) food habits or behaviors, (2) knowledge or achievement gain, and (3) attitudes.

Behavior Change—Conceptual and Methodological Aspects

Behavior change is probably the major controversy in nutrition education and in the evaluation of nutrition education programs. The real measure of effective nutrition education is a change not in knowledge or attitude but in behavior, as well as maintenance of existing desirable behaviors. Such alterations in any area are difficult to achieve. We have only to look at the widespread campaign to decrease smoking in the American population; after several years, this debilitating habit is beginning to show a decrease.

Those who are not closely involved with the problem of achieving behavorial change are demanding evidence that dollars spent on programs are achieving the intended behavioral changes. Frequently, such evidence is demanded after only three or four weeks of nutrition education, or at the extremes of generosity, after six months or a year. Until controversy over the amount of time and effort required to realize behavioral change is resolved, issues concerning the design and conduct of evaluation projects will remain confounded.

Kolbe states that "without behavioral analysis we cannot determine whether our programs are effective in eliciting appropriate behaviors, let alone how to design such programs to be more effective" (1979, p. 12). In assessing the effectiveness of various health education programs applicable to nutrition education, Kolbe outlines problems intrinsic to the use of behavioral criteria. Most of the points are characteristic of health education programs, not of behavioral research. These programs attempt to influence many different and unrelated behaviors, are addressed to fairly large groups, and focus primarily upon a youthful population. He believes that it is difficult to observe health–related behaviors and, furthermore, to determine whether or not these behaviors are the result of specific educational programs. In addition, teachers are not trained in the use of evaluation methodologies and sometimes feel threatened by evaluation efforts. He argues that English and history, for example, are not evaluated on the short-term basis often applied to health education programs. Another confounding aspect of evaluating behavorial change is the focus on the consequence without providing answers as to why or why not programs are effective. Kolbe is concerned that this kind of focus, although

a necessary part of education evaluation, can push education toward a persuasion or communication technique approach. He believes that all the problems he outlines are even more intense at
the elementary school level than at upper levels.

Education is not the only factor leading to behavior change, but
other significant factors are extremely difficult to define or measure in research and evaluation studies. Behavior change must be
considered in a broad context that includes ethnicity, geographic
location, available technology, and economic situation (Lowenberg
1974), and a great number of variables influence food behavior
(Rand 1976). Acceptance of change is influenced by familiarity
with food, early childhood experiences with foods, self-image, trau-
matic experiences related to food, literacy, and certain personality
characteristics such as rigidity or anxiety. A student's awareness
of all these influences enhances the effectiveness of nutrition education programs.

Without an adequate working definition of behavior change, we
sometimes look for such change in the wrong ways or use incorrect
criteria or measurement instruments. Paradoxically, we often ig-
nore obvious indicators of behavior change, perhaps because they
are so obvious. For example, much evidence indicates people today
are more interested in health and nutrition than in previous
decades. Health food stores are staying in business, jogging shoes
are selling, consumption of certain foods thought to be causally
related to various diseases has decreased, and citizen pressure on
the federal government has led to increased support of nutrition
research, education, and policy. These trends would seem to indicate behavior change. We will never know if this behavior change
is a result of nutrition education alone, but such education may be
one impetus for change.

Probably some of the best writing about the nutritional status
of people has been done on the topic of food habits or food behaviors, initiated by works of Margaret Mead during the Second World
War. Primarily, the thinking has evolved around discussions of
which variables constituted food behaviors or habits and the need
to develop effective nutrition education programs. In discussing
the problems of food habit research, Mead wrote:

  Early in our work on food habits it became evident that there
  was a need for a code that would make possible a formal

description of a people's dietary pattern. Such a code would allow for the description of food in all its different aspects:
1. In psychological sensory terms . . .
2. In terms of its chemistry . . .
3. In nutritional terms . . .
4. In cultural terms . . .
    a. agricultural . . .
    b. economic . . .
    c. socio-cultural . . .
    d. educational . . .
    e. related to food handling . . .
    f. related to dietary patterning . . . (1964, p. 22).

Mead held that unless such a formal code for describing and recording patterns of food habits was developed, the science of this field would stay ". . . essentially what it is today—a fragmented set of associations casually related to the relevant disciplines" (1964, p. 23). No such formal code has been adopted, and the result is as Mead anticipated—the field remains fragmented, and interdisciplinary efforts are infrequent and awkward.

Grivetti and Pangborn (1973) focused on the need for nutrition educators to recognize existing food habits, especially from a cultural perspective. The researchers reviewed and critiqued seven foci important when collecting data on food habits: environment, cultural ecology, region, culture and history, functionalism, quantity, and clinical characteristics. They believed that several factors combined provided the information important to nutrition educators eager to develop exciting new dimensions of food habits.

Yetley (1974) used the techniques of causal modeling and path analysis to identify relationships among variables which relate to human food behaviors. In this work, she applied the philosophies of Mead and others to study food behaviors from multiple standpoints.

For the last thirty years, these authors have urged educators to think of food habits as a multivariate concept, but the methodology has often been narrow in scope, predominantly restricted to recall and recording of foods eaten. While studies often use this recall technique and report data without any discussion of the limitations involved, the validity of the information about what people are eating is questionable (Madden, Goodman, and Guthrie 1976; Gersovitz, Madden, and Smiciklas–Wright 1978; Emmons and Hayes 1973). People tend to report what they believe is socially acceptable behavior, rather than actual behavior; small intakes are often over–reported and large intakes under–reported. In behavior change studies which use control groups, a possible outcome is the underestimation of the effectiveness of a nutrition program in improving low intakes or decreasing excessive ones. Although some studies report similar results from twenty-four hour recalls as from seven-day-or-longer records, other studies do not always agree, suggesting that accuracy begins to decline after the fifth or sixth day.

Another study used regression equations with three–day food records to predict nutritional adequacy of the diet, with a reliability of 80 percent; the researchers concluded: "A relatively small number of foods seems to provide enough information about diets to make predictions about their nutrient adequacy" (Johnson and Schwinn 1979, p. 107). They warned, however, that the regression coefficients they developed were population–specific and needed constant reevaluation.

Huenemann (1971) emphasized that short-term (that is, twenty-four-hour and three-day) dietary intake does not necessarily measure nutritional status. Evaluators must look at other factors as well, because teenagers in particular vary in their daily nutrient consumption.

Results of another study also indicate the need for caution in interpreting data. In this study of elementary school children and their parents, the researchers found ". . . that these three variables are independent of one another and should not be used interchangeably to represent food habits when evaluating the effectiveness of nutrition education programs . . ." (Yperman and Vermeersch 1979, p. 72).

Controversy surrounding the criteria used to analyze food records data has arisen, with many researchers avoiding the limited "Basic Four" or major nutrient approach and turning to broader criteria. One recently used technique is the index of nutritional quality (INQ), based on the nutrients in a food quantity that contains x number of calories divided by the Recommended Daily Allowances (RDA) of those nutrients (Abdel-Ghany 1978).

Knowledge

Studies which evaluate the effectiveness of various nutrition education programs usually include a statement such as: "A knowledge test was developed and administered." Often these measurement instruments are specific to the particular study, with little or no information given about how they were developed, piloted, validated, and administered; their soundness or adaptability are difficult to judge.

With the current emphasis on nutrition education, tests are becoming available nationally for a variety of situations; however, many fail to list complete information about the test's development and characteristics.

There exist a few test reviews, such as Buros's *Mental Measurement Yearbooks* (1978), which focus on a variety of information: test reliability, how content validation was achieved, what learning objectives served as the base for question development, how extensively the tests were piloted, and mean scores or norms. Unfortunately, these data often are not available for nutrition education instruments, perhaps because of the brief history of test development in this area and the failure of educators to work closely with test and measurement consultants.

One commercially available nutrition test is called *The Nutrition Assessment Inventory* (NTS Research Corporation 1978). The introductory materials describe this test as measuring knowledge, attitude, and behavior. There are separate paper-and-pencil tests for primary, intermediate, junior high, and senior high school students and adults. However, there are pitfalls. The test is listed as developed by a team of authors recognized as experts in nutrition education and measurement; no names or affiliations are listed. A three-year development process involving content analysis of many materials and programs is claimed; no programs are identified. Information is not provided concerning piloting, content validation, or reliability. NTS Research Corporation analyzes the student data on completed answer sheets; no keys giving correct answers are provided in the test manual.

The test's behavior questions seem broad, including such examples as "Do you eat breakfast every day?" to which a "yes/no" response is requested, or "Do you eat a lot of candy and cookies?" The attitude section consists of statements with which students are to agree or disagree, or, in the later tests for intermediate and junior high school, to select from "always/most of the time/sometimes/or never." Although requested, information concerning the cost of the tests and the cost of providing data analysis services was not made available to the reviewer.

The *Nutrition Education Assessment Series* includes a complete series of tests for schoolchildren (Planning, Development and Evaluation Associates, Inc. 1979). Test development is described to some extent, but the nutrition educators involved are not identified. The paper–pencil tests are said to focus on knowledge, attitudes, and habits. The tests were printed for distribution and sale at the same time they were prepared for pilot testing; therefore, reliability data and norms were not available until recently. Concurrent and construct validity is to develop over time, according to the authors, as further studies are conducted. This test development process illustrates perhaps the unique approach resulting from the pressures for measurement instruments in an area where few are available.*

Pennsylvania State University (1979a, 1980), in its extensive curriculum development project, has also included achievement test development. Separate tests exist for kindergarten, grades one through three, four, five, and six. These tests are tied to the units of instruction in the curriculum, "Nutrition in a Changing World," and are available from the Nutrition Foundation for $3.00 each. There are also nutrition examinations for teachers taking an in-service college course for credit. The items are well written and have been thoroughly validated by nutritionists. Statistical evidence to describe test characteristics is available (Pennsylvania State University 1979b).

The Dairy Council Inc.'s basic, easily analyzed achievement test, used as a pre- and post-test with second and sixth grades in some of their evaluation projects, focuses on knowledge of the Basic Four food groups and serving sizes (Dairy Council Inc. of California 1974). This test could be used for measuring specific learning situa-

---

*Copies are available at $1.00 each. PDE also provides a useful service: for $.60 per test, they will machine-score the tests and provide a performance summary for a district; for $.80 per test, they will have it machine-scored and provide an individual student report; for $.25 per test, PDE will scan but not conduct the analysis of each test.

tions in the lower grades. There are no data available on test reliability, difficulty, or norms.

An achievement test which does provide a description of its development process and statistics about reliability, discriminability, difficulty levels, and some average scores achieved by students taking the exam is available from the National Dairy Council (1979). The *Nutrition Achievement Test: K–6* was initially developed for the evaluation work related to the *FOOD . . . Your Choice* nutrition education program. An Iowa State University research team collected extensive item analysis data to revise the test, further study content and construct validity, and develop information about reliability, difficulty, discriminability, and mean scores. The content of the test is built around the White House Conference concepts, which are clearly outlined and identified in the test manual. Available from local Dairy Council offices or the National Dairy Council, the material is printed as a package, with an accompanying test manual and three separate tests: one for kindergarten through grade two, one for grades three and four, and one for grades five and six. Teachers are permitted to make multiple copies of the test master for classroom use.

A 1975 nutrition knowledge test for elementary school teachers was developed at Pennsylvania State University as a precursor to later instruments. Described as especially valuable in needs assessments for teacher training programs, the test is composed of two parts: the first contains statements requiring true/false responses, each with a degree of certainty response; and the second consists of selected short paragraphs from the lay nutrition literature requiring various responses. This tool is one of the few instruments for which a journal article on development and test characteristics is available (Carver and Lewis 1979). The authors suggest that the test can be especially valuable in needs assessments for teacher training programs.

Lindsey (1973) reported on a unique approach to the development of instruments. An instrument, developed to evaluate the nutrition objectives of a 4-H day camp in Minnesota for eight to ten year olds, consisted of a twelve-key electrical wiring board; the designers believed that students at this age would have difficulty with a written device. The instrument was piloted with a group of eight and nine year olds to determine ease of use and level of understanding. No other description of development was given.

Several other instruments used in reported research studies are available from the various authors, including a test for teacher in-service education, composed of true/false and multiple choice questions focusing on knowledge. The journal article gives no description of instrument development (Grogan 1978).

Another test, "The Teenage Nutrition Survey," includes a twenty-four-hour recall sheet, thirty food habit questions, queries about likes and dislikes, and ten multiple choice items related to knowledge. With a reported reliability index of KR–20 = .42, the multiple choice items were ". . . checked for validity by two nutrition instructors . . ." (Axelson and Del Campo 1978, p. 30). This instrument was used for a mass media study.

Eppright et al. (1970) developed a nutrition knowledge test for use with mothers participating in a North Central regional study of diets. In the preliminary development, nutritionists selected and scored true/false statements relating to nutrition knowledge, food composition, food misconceptions, and the application of principles of nutrition. After deleting ambiguous items, the authors used the thirty-five most highly intercorrelated items in the final knowledge test. Although the test format is true/false, there is also a "don't know" category and a section to indicate one of five degrees of certainty for each response.

Attitude

Very few instruments, particularly at the elementary school level, have been developed to measure attitudes related to the area of nutrition. Head et al. (1974) describe an instrument for measuring student attitudes toward selected school factors, one subscale of which is related to the School Lunch Program. The subscale contains thirty-eight items and offers a choice of one of five responses, ranging from strongly agree to strongly disagree. According to the description of scale development, the scale was piloted after validation by a jury drawn from education and food service fields to develop standardization. Following administration to 2,785 students, the tests were analyzed, revised, and reoffered. Unfortunately, one version was used as the pretest and another version as the posttest, a troubling situation when it is not clear exactly what kinds of revisions were made. The description mentions that the pretest data were rescored in view of the posttest changes. Both reliability and intercorrelations of items in the six subscales are reported.

The instrument developed by Eppright et al. (1970) contains an attitude scale, as well as the knowledge test described in the previous section. Statements derived from interviews and open-ended questionnaires were used to develop the attitude scale used in this research. Then homemaker responses to the statements made in a pilot test were analyzed to select the most highly intercorrelated items for the final scales. Possible responses were "agree" or "disagree" and "favorable" or "unfavorable," with the degree of certainty indicated. These instruments were then used in a study of nutrition knowledge, attitudes, and practices four years after graduation of high school students who had had a home economics course. This is one of the few semilongitudinal studies found in the literature (Schwartz 1975).

The only instruments located which focused on school food service personnel were a set used at Kansas State University. These were developed and sent to school food service personnel to determine attitudes and information about their program activities. The instruments did not focus on knowledge, nor was information about their development and use available (Hallet 1977).

EVALUATION STUDIES OF SCHOOL PROGRAMS

Since most studies in this review focus on a particular program or a curriculum in a specific setting, their applicability cannot be generalized nor can their program effectiveness be classified as either research or evaluation. We believe that such a fine-lined distinction is not critical, because both research and evaluation guide the design and methodology of future evaluation studies.

The studies are reviewed primarily from the standpoint of design and instrumentation, with no attempt made to describe the results, as this is not the section's purpose. (Later chapters detail content in regard to students, teachers, and school food service personnel.) The following studies are reviewed in four sections: elementary school programs, secondary school programs, those involving the school food service, and those involving teachers.

Elementary School Programs

Baker (1972) conducted a carefully designed experiment which looked at physical, attitudinal, and dietary characteristics and knowledge scores of 200 students in a program in which thirteen thirty-minute lessons had been taught. Development of the knowledge test was thoroughly described, although the text was not piloted with large numbers of students, and there were no reports on reliability. Height, weight, skin fold, and arm and leg girth data were collected to describe physical characteristics. A hedonic scale, gathering information about attitudes toward vegetables, was developed and used. In terms of behavior, two twenty-four-hour food recalls and one twenty-four-hour food record, pre- and post-test, were used with both experimental and control groups.

Looking at cognitive behavioral changes of fourth and fifth graders, Wang and Dwyer (1975) adapted questionnaires used by Abt Associates Inc. to evaluate a nationwide nutrition education program; the researchers modified questions for Chinese food habits and translated them into Chinese for administration. All procedures and statistical work were clearly and thoroughly explained.

Talmage et al. (1978) reported on the summative evaluation of the kindergarten through sixth grade *FOOD . . . Your Choice* program, conducted by the Office of Evaluation Research at the University of Illinois, Chicago Circle. In this report, the test development process and statistical characteristics are not described; such information is available from the authors. The study gathered data about knowledge, learning environment, attitude, and behavior, but it is particularly useful because of the authors' thorough discussion of its unique design and procedures. For example, the design permitted a satisfactory solution to the issue of control groups. Often it is difficult to justify the selection of some students to serve as controls because of the feeling that all students should benefit from a good experience. Therefore, this design called for a control group in the fall; in the spring this group participated in the nutrition education program. The design also provided for data collection at three different times—pre-, mid-, and post-study —that would not otherwise have been possible.

In evaluating the U.S. Department of Agriculture's television program, "Mulligan Stew," Abt Associates Inc. had three major purposes: (1) evaluate the impact of the program on student learning; (2) describe, through case studies, specific planning and training efforts used to implement the program in selected sites; and (3) conduct a content analysis of the films from the two standpoints of production value and specific nutritional content. Thoroughly designed instruments were presented in the final report and appear to have been given considerable attention during development (Shapiro, Bale, and Scardino 1974). However, the specific development process for these instruments is not described in the four-volume report of the study. Both this study and that by the University of Illinois for the National Dairy Council are examples of the many components included in sound national evaluations of major educational programs.

A well-designed study of much smaller scale contains a thorough discussion of instrument development, including a knowledge test, a vegetable preference rating scale, and a luncheon habits questionnaire (Smith and Justice 1979). The knowledge test was validated by third grade teachers for content readability and appropriateness and by a professor of nutrition for content validity, and the report lists discriminability, difficulty, and reliability statistics. An interesting aspect of this study is the fact that the researcher taught all the nutrition lessons, thereby controlling for teacher variation but leaving open the question of whether the results are attributable to the program or to the instructor.

Several other studies made little or no mention of the procedures used to develop the various test instruments, a point illustrated by the following comments: "The content validity was assured by basing the test items on the behavioral objectives specified in *Big Ideas Module*" (Bell and Lamb 1973, p. 197). "A test of nutrition knowledge consisting of 37 multiple choice or fill-in questions was developed and administered to the students . . ." (Jenkins, Stumo, and Voichick 1975, p. 17). Cosper, Hayslip, and Foree (1977) mention that the validity of their test was checked against the grid of behavioral objectives and that each objective was covered in at least two test items. Tolin et al. (1979) similarly describe the items on their test as being evaluated for validity and readability by two education professors. In studies by Shovic and Jennings (1979), Boysen and Ahrens (1972), and Head et al. (1974), little mention is made of the type of tests used or their development.

Other studies can be critiqued in terms of methodology and manner of data reporting. Two reporters talk of their procedure: "It was not deemed necessary to assess comparison classes that had no nutrition in the program. Gains were expected to be substantial, and it was believed highly unlikely that uninstructed pupils would make gains similar to those of the instructed groups during the two or three weeks required for the tryouts" (Niedermeyer and Moncreif 1975, p. 307). In this study, a fourteen-item pretest and a twenty-eight-item posttest were used to measure knowledge gains. Why the tests were of two different lengths and how this affected analysis of data are unclear in the report. All data were in terms of percent gain from the fourteen-item to the twenty-eight-item test, and were also analyzed in terms of various socioeconomic and ethnic classifications.

Lovett, Barker, and Marcus, in an earlier study of the same nutrition education program, chose Los Angeles as their only test site ". . . because it offered typical, reliable, projectable results" (1970, p. 81). They reported a 360 percent increase for the experimental group versus 51 and 76 percent for the two semicontrol groups (in one teachers received materials only, in the other they received materials and some general health education objectives). Although they mentioned that these data were verified by accepted statistical measures to qualify the high results, no statistical data were reported.

Secondary School Programs

In another study in which the goal was to assess general level of knowledge and interest in nutrition, there is a thorough discussion of test development. A one-hundred-item nutrition knowledge questionnaire was developed and thoroughly reviewed by a panel of experts in a study of content validity. Construct validation processes, difficulty, discriminability characteristics, and other data were reported (Dwyer, Feldman, and Mayer 1970).

Picardi and Porter (1976) describe the content, length, reliability, item difficulty, and discriminability of their nutrition knowledge tests used to measure high school students' knowledge before and after a food and nutrition minicourse in both experimental and control classrooms. This study also used an attitude test which employed a ranking technique. In the test, eight nutrition-related health problems were presented by pairs in random order; the respondents checked the problem in each pair which concerned them more. The same approach was used with eight food choice behaviors, the respondents selecting the one behavior from each pair which better described how they chose foods for a meal. Procedures included a study of the correlations among the three factors of knowledge, attitude, and behavior.

A study by Podell et al. (1978) is interesting because the researchers included a biochemical test in the evaluation design. Before and after a cardiovascular nutrition education program, serum cholesterol levels were measured. These and other studies (Palgi et al. 1976, Axelson and DelCampo 1978) focus on knowledge, attitudes, and eating behavior in discussing effective nutrition education programs. However, no studies describe the procedures used to develop various instruments for gathering data on these three factors.

School Food Service

A major aspect of the Nutrition Education and Training Program legislation is the relationship between the school food service program and other aspects of nutrition education in the school. Several research and evaluation studies which incorporate school food service are treated in this section of the paper. Again, the studies are reviewed from the standpoint of design and instrumentation as a guide toward future development.

An extensive study of school food service–based nutrition education programs involved the development of curriculum materials and evaluation instruments, as well as the implementation and evaluation phases. However, the researchers provide a sketchy description of the evaluation instrument development process: ". . . the knowledge tests as well as all of the instruments were age-appropriate, having been developed by project staff and reviewed by a project consultant experienced in instrument design. Reading level verifications were used on all instruments employing the Fry Test of Readability" (O'Brien et al. 1976, p. 326). The researchers failed to indicate whether the project staff were qualified to judge age appropriateness, whether the content was reviewed by subject matter experts, and whether the instruments were pilot tested.

Studying photographs of plate waste and measuring food are techniques used in several studies. Garrett and Vaden (1978) examined the influence of student-selected menus on elementary students' lunch program participation, plate waste, and attitudes toward school food service. Although they used instruments to measure attitude and food preference, they failed to describe the development process for either instrument.

Herzog et al. (1978) studied the use of informal teaching techniques in a high school lunch program—table tents and wall posters—in affecting students' knowledge, food consumption, and plate waste. Pre- and post-test data were collected, but there was no discussion of the development of the eighteen–item knowledge test or the food consumption instrument, except to report that the focus was on students' selection of "more nutritional" items.

Evans and Vaden (1979) used several data-gathering approaches to study the effect of student advisory councils on school food service programs. The council activities were listed, and members were asked to rank activities on a five-point scale ranging from very worthwhile to not worthwhile. Student attitudes toward the food service program before and after the six-month period of council operation were gathered using an adaptation of an instrument described in earlier studies. Each study day, the percent of the lunch program participants in school was calculated.

To help identify variables in school food service programs which influenced food choices, Talmage and Iverson (1979) chose the case study approach. According to the approach, future work in evaluation and research studies will be most valuable if a variety of factors are examined: attitudes of school food service personnel, physical facilities, the color and attractiveness of walls and tables in the school lunch room, and the flexibility of the menu.

Teachers

Most evaluation studies in nutrition education which examine data gathered from teachers focus on teacher preservice and inservice education; a few evaluations focus on the teachers of these programs. We reviewed both types of studies.

A unique Canadian study attempted to tie together the changes among the students that could be reasonably attributed to a teacher education workshop on nutrition and use of certain curricular materials (Cooper and Philp 1974). Teachers assessed the achievement and claimed behavior of the students by asking what they had had for breakfast the day of the test. A second purpose of the study was to determine, through teacher reports, the number of teachers who implemented the nutrition education program in their classrooms following the workshop and the extent to which they covered the objectives. There was no assessment of knowledge gain or attitude change on the part of the teachers.

A project at Eastern Washington State University attempted to encourage future elementary teachers to include nutrition education in their programs (Stronck 1976). Funded by the National Dairy Council, the project developed a model for preparing these students to teach nutrition by incorporating nutrition education into several existing courses in reading, literature, language arts, and educational psychology. The focus of the evaluation was on attitudinal change, as reflected by questionnaire responses administered after presentations on nutrition topics in the various courses.

Grogan (1978) constructed an innovative, three-part study to evaluate teachers who planned to incorporate nutrition in existing curricula. In studying this inservice program, which consisted of courses in nutrition and teaching methods, Grogan first administered a fifty-item multiple choice and true/false test both before and after the program. There is no mention of how the test was developed. The second part of the evaluation focused on the degree to which the teachers believed the course objectives had been successfully accomplished. Following the course, trained nutrition educators visited classrooms to observe the degree of success teachers were having in implementing the integrated curriculum. The third part of this study involved the pre- and post-testing of a representative sample of 300 students of these teachers, using the same test as in the first part.

Several studies of the nutrition education programs conducted by the National Dairy Council have looked to teachers as sources of evaluation data about elementary nutrition education programs. Talmage and Rasher (1978b) conducted a study to determine whether students and teachers who had used a specific nutrition education program differed from other students and teachers (in the same school building and in other schools in the district) not using the curriculum. The methodology involved administration of a short interview of ten questions to groups of teachers in each of these three settings. There was no report discussion of the procedures used to develop the questionnaire. The same authors in another study focused on the follow-up aspects of curriculum implementation, specifically, how teachers using the program for two years differed from those using it only one year (Talmage and Rasher 1978a). Again teachers were interviewed to gather data on their ratings of the curriculum materials, the amount of additional training they felt was necessary for successful implementation of nutrition education programs, clarity of materials, use of student worksheets, and the degree to which they saw positive behavioral changes in their students.

A study conducted for the Dairy, Food and Nutrition Council of Minnesota (1976) used a mailed questionnaire. There was no clear discussion of the purposes of the study nor of the development of the questionnaire. The study compared teachers who had received inservice training in the use of a nutrition education program with teachers who had not, and looked at differences in the groups' perceptions of the importance of nutrition education, satisfaction with Dairy Council materials, degree of comfort in teaching nutrition, and degree to which each shared with others ideas and information about teaching nutrition.

Carruth and Musgrave (1979) used a semantic differential approach for determining changes in attitude following a college-level community nutrition course. Twenty-five bipolar adjective scales were used in what the authors described as a quantifiable tool to measure attitude changes about nutrition education. There was no extensive discussion of the development of the instrument.

CONCLUSION

Most evaluation studies of school programs use experimental and control groups, most use a pre- and post-testing design, and some also employ retention. The majority of studies imply that some attention has been given to the development of the various instruments used but fail to describe development in the detail required to provide the reader with solid criteria for evaluating the data. Little mention is made of school and teacher variables, Hawthorne effects, or other problems and issues. Some researchers are trying innovative designs and procedures to help answer the complex questions of nutrition education effectiveness.

Evaluation in nutrition education has passed from infancy into adolescence. Except for a few missing pieces, the strategies and models of evaluation are ready to be applied rigorously in studying the effectiveness of nutrition education in school settings, as well as in community and clinical environments. The current task is to fill in these missing pieces. We must concentrate efforts in several areas:

1. Clarify the purposes of nutrition education to guide the focus of evaluation. This needs to occur at several levels within the profession, within the federal government, and at state, local, and program levels.

2. Define and conceptualize critical terms upon which evaluation designs rely, such as "behavior change," "food habits," "attitudes," "nutritious," and "adequate knowledge." Definition of such terms is critical to focusing the purposes of nutrition education and guiding evaluation.

3. Develop instrumentation that will describe and measure the stated and the true outcomes of nutrition education. We do not currently have a bank of instruments from which to draw, nor do we find reports of adequate procedures in the design of instruments used in current studies.

4. Use designs appropriate to the evaluation questions asked.

5. Provide education and support to nutrition educators and others who are expected to conduct evaluation studies. It is unrealistic to expect all nutrition educators and others supporting their programs to conduct large-scale evaluations. However, evaluation on a smaller and continuous basis by those conducting programs can provide immediate feedback for program improvement and decision making.

6. Conduct research studies to answer the questions we have in nutrition education. For example, we need research to develop instruments, to study the effects of measurement itself on various food behaviors, and to achieve professional consensus on certain issues, including terminology.

7. Communicate and use the results of evaluation studies to build the theoretical and conceptual framework for evaluation and for nutrition education.

8.   Educate administrators and policymakers about realistic
     expectations and procedures for evaluation in nutrition
     education.

Evaluation of nutrition education is a complex process confounded by unresolved issues and undeveloped strategies. However, we
are now at a point of development and interest in both evaluation
and nutrition education at which major progress can be made.

BIBLIOGRAPHY

Abdel-Ghany, M. 1978. Evaluation of Household Diets by the Index of Nutritional Quality. *J. Nutr. Educ.* 10:79.

American Dietetic Association. 1973. Position Paper on Nutrition Education for the Public. *J. Am. Dietet. Assoc.* 62:429.

———. 1974. Position Paper on Child Nutrition Programs. *J. Am. Dietet. Assoc.* 64:520.

———. 1978. Position Paper on the Scope and Thrust of Nutrition Education. *J. Am. Dietet. Assoc.* 72:302.

Austin, J.E. 1978. The Perilous Journey of Nutrition Evaluation. *Am. J. Clin. Nutr.* 31:2324.

Axelson, J.M., and DelCampo, D.S. 1978. Improving Teenagers' Nutrition Knowledge through the Mass Media. *J. Nutr. Educ.* 10:30.

Baker, M.J. 1972. Influence of Nutrition Education on Fourth and Fifth Graders. *J. Nutr. Educ.* 4:55.

Bell, C.G., and Lamb, M.W. 1973. Nutrition Education and Dietary Behavior of Fifth Graders. *J. Nutr. Educ.* 5:196.

Bloom, B.I.; Hastings, J.T.; and Madaus, G.F. 1971. *Handbook on Formative and Summative Evaluation of Student Learning.* New York: McGraw-Hill.

Borg, W.R., and Gall, M.D. 1979. *Educational Research: An Introduction.* 3rd ed. New York: Longman.

Boysen, S.C., and Ahrens, R.A. 1972. Nutrition Instruction and Lunch Surveys with Second Graders. *J. Nutr. Educ.* 4:172.

Buros, Oscar K. 1978. *Eighth Mental Measurement Yearbook.* Highland Park, N.J.: Gryphon Press.

Campbell, D.R., and Stanley, J. 1973. *Experimental and Quasi-Experimental Designs for Research.* Chicago: Rand McNally.

Carruth, B.R., and Musgrave, K.O. 1979. Changing Attitudes in Community Nutrition. *J. Nutr. Educ.* 11:127.

Carver, L., and Lewis, K. 1979. A Nutrition Knowledge Test for Elementary School Teachers. *J. Nutr. Educ.* 11:68.

Cooper, B., and Philp, M. 1974. Evaluation of Nutrition Education in Everyday Teaching Environment. *J. Nutr. Educ.* 6:99.

Cooper, K.A., and Go, C.E. 1976. Analyses of Nutrition Curriculum Guides at the K–12 Level. *J. Nutr. Educ.* 8:62.

Cosper, B.A.; Hayslip, D.E.; and Foree, S.B. 1977. The Effect of

Nutrition Education on Dietary Habits of Fifth Graders. *J. Sch. Health* 47:475.

Dairy Council of California. 1974. *Pretest and Posttest—Daily Food Choices.* Sacramento: Dairy Council of California.

Dairy, Food and Nutrition Council of Minnesota. 1976. *An Evaluation of the Educational Materials and Big Ideas Workshop of the Dairy, Food and Nutrition Council of Minnesota.* St. Paul, Minn., October 1976.

Dwyer, J.T.; Feldman, J.J.; and Mayer, J. 1970. Nutritional Literacy of High School Students. *J. Nutr. Educ.* 2:59.

Eash, M.J., and Rasher, S.P. 1976. *A Needs Assessment of Nutrition Education.* Office of Evaluation Research. Chicago: University of Illinois at Chicago Circle.

Eash, M.J. et al. 1977. Report on the Field Tests of the National Dairy Council's Nutrition Education. 3 vols. Technical Report 89. Office of Evaluation Research. Chicago: University of Illinois at Chicago Circle.

Emmons, L., and Hayes, M. 1973. Accuracy of 24-Hour Recalls of Young Children. *J. Am. Dietet. Assoc.* 62:409.

Eppright, E.S. 1970. Nutrition Knowledge and Attitudes of Mothers (The North Central Regional Study of Diets of Preschool Children). *J. Home Econ.* 62:327.

Evans, S.K., and Vaden, A.G. 1979. Evaluation of Student Advisory Councils for School Food Service Programs. *School Food Service Res. Rev.* 3:85.

Foley, C.; Hertzler, A.A.; and Anderson, H.L. 1979. Attitudes and Food Habits—A Review. *J. Am. Dietet. Assoc.* 75:13.

Fruin, M.F., and Davison, M.L. 1978. Some Considerations in the Measurement of Change. *J. Am. Dietet. Assoc.* 73:15.

Garrett, P.W., and Vaden, A.G. 1978. Influence of Student–Selected Menus on Participation, Plate Waste, and Student Attitudes. *School Food Service Res. Rev.* 2:28.

Gersovitz, M.; Madden, J.P.; and Smiciklas-Wright, H. 1978. Validity of the 24-Hour Dietary Recall and Seven-Day Record for Group Comparisons. *J. Am. Dietet. Assoc.* 73:48.

Green, L.W. 1977. Evaluation and Measurement: Some Dilemmas for Health Education, *Am. J. Pub. Health.* 67:155.

Grivetti, L.E., and Pangborn, R.M. 1973. Food Habit Research: A Review of Approaches and Methods. *J. Nutr. Educ.* 5:204.

Grogan, J. 1978. Teacher Inservice for Nutrition Education—An

Interdisciplinary Approach in the School System. *J. Nutr. Educ.* 10:119.

Gronlund, N.E. 1976. *Measurement and Evaluation in Teaching.* 3rd ed. New York: Macmillan.

Guthrie, H.A. 1977. Concept of a Nutritious Food. *J. Am. Dietet. Assoc.* 71:14.

―――. 1978. Is Education Not Enough? *J. Nutr. Educ.* 10:57.

Hallet, S.G. 1977. Administrators and Public Policy: Implications for the School Food Service Program. Unpublished Master's thesis, Kansas State University.

Head, M.K. et al. 1974. A Scale for Measuring Student Attitudes Toward Selected School Factors. *Ed. and Psych. Measur.* 34:971.

Hertzler, A.A., and Owen, C. 1974. Sociologic Study of Food Habits: A Review. *J. Am. Dietet. Assoc.* 69:381.

Herzog, L.J. et al. 1978. Evaluation of an Informal Nutrition Education Approach in a High School Lunch Program. *School Food Service Res. Rev.* 2:102.

Hochbaum, G.M. 1977. Human Behavior and Nutrition Education. *Nutrition News* 40:1.

Huenemann, R.L. 1971. A Review of Teenage Nutrition in the United States. In *Proceedings of National Nutrition Education Conference.* Pub. no. 1254: 37. Washington, D.C.: U.S. Department of Agriculture.

Jenkins, S.; Stumo, M.; and Voichick, J. 1975. Evaluation of the Nutrition Film Series "Mulligan Stew." *J. Nutr. Educ.* 7:17.

Johnson, N.E., and Schwinn, S. 1978. Coefficients for Estimation of Nutrient Adequacy Scores of Diets of a Specific Population Group. *Home Ec. Res. J.* 7:98.

Kolbe, L. 1979. Evaluating Effectiveness—The Problems of Behavioral Criteria. *Health Educ.* (Jan/Feb 1979):12.

Levine, R.R.; McChesney, A.S.; and Brush, M.K. 1979. An Assessment of High School Nutrition Education. *J. Nutr. Educ.* 11:124.

Light, L. 1978. Nutrition Education: Policies and Programs. *Nutrition Program News.* Washington, D.C.: U.S. Department of Agriculture (Jan–April).

Lindsey, D.E. 1973. Evaluating Nutrition Teaching. *Extension Serv. Rev.* (Sept/Oct 1973):3.

Lovett, R.; Barker, E.; and Marcus, B. 1970. The Effect of a Nutrition Education Program at the Second Grade Level, *J. Nutr. Educ.* 2:Supp. 1.

Lowenberg, M.E. 1974. The Development of Food Behavior. *J. Am. Dietet. Assoc.* 65:263.

Madden, J.P.; Goodman, S.J.; and Guthrie, H.A. 1976. Validity of the 24-Hour Recall. *J. Am. Dietet. Assoc.* 68:143.

Mapes, M.C. 1977. GULP—An Alternate Method for Teaching Teens. *J. Nutr. Educ.* 9:12.

Maretzki, A.N. 1979a. A Comparison of Curriculum Planning Methodologies for Nutrition Education, K–12. Paper presented at the annual meeting of the American Education Research Association, San Francisco, April.

————. 1979b. A Perspective on Nutrition Education and Training. *J. Nutr. Educ.* 11:176.

McCool, A.C. 1979. Program Evaluation for Effective Resource Management and Accountability. *J. Am. Dietet. Assoc.* 75:564.

McKenzie, J.C., and Mumford, P. 1965. The Evaluation of Nutrition Education Programmes: A Review of the Present Situation. *World Review of Nutrition and Dietetics* 5:21.

Mead, M. 1964. Food Habits Research: Problems of the 1960s. Pub. 1225. Washington, D.C.: National Academy of Sciences, National Research Council.

Morris, L., and Fitz-Gibbon, C.J. 1978. *Evaluator's Handbook.* Beverly Hills: Sage.

National Dairy Council. 1979. *The Nutrition Achievement Test: K–6.* Chicago: National Dairy Council.

Niedermeyer, F.C., and Moncrief, M.H. 1975. Primary Graders Study Nutrition. *Elem. Schl. J.* 75:305.

NTS Research Corporation. 1978. *The Nutrition Assessment Inventory.* Durham, N.C.: NTS Research Corporation.

O'Brien, R.E. et al. 1976. Comprehensive School Food Service–Related Nutrition Education Curriculum Evaluation Project Grades K–12, Final Report, Part I: Study Design and Results. Silver Spring, Maryland: Applied Management Sciences.

Olson, J.C., and Sims, L. 1980. Assessing Nutrition Knowledge from an Information Processing Perspective. *J. Nutr. Educ.* 12:157.

Palgi, A. et al. 1976. Body Weight as a Health Index: A Minicourse in Nutrition. *J. Nutr. Educ.* 8:126.

Pennsylvania State University. 1979a. *Nutrition Knowledge Test for Nursery and Kindergarten and Nutrition Knowledge Test: Primary Grades 1–3.* Washington, D.C.: Nutrition Foundation.

————. 1979b. *Teacher Nutrition Questions.* University Park, Penn.: Pennsylvania State University.

————. 1980. *Nutrition Challenge I–1, Nutrition Challenge I–2, and Nutrition Challenge I–3.* University Park, Penn.: Pennsylvania State University.

Picardi, S., and Porter, D. 1976. Multidimensional Evaluation of a Food and Nutrition Minicourse. *J. Nutr. Educ.* 8:162.

Planning, Development and Evaluation Associates, Inc. 1979. *Nutrition Education Series.* Tampa, Florida: PDEA, Inc.

Podell, R.N. et al. 1978. Evaluation of the Effectiveness of a High School Course in Cardiovascular Nutrition. *Am. J. Pub. Health* 68:573.

Ramsey, C.E., and Cloyd, M. 1979. Multiple Objectives and the Success of Educational Programs. *J. Nutr. Educ.* 11:141.

Rand, C. 1976. Nutrition Behavior: Exploring Its Sociological Influences. *Ill. Teacher* 19:198.

Reaburn, J.A.; Krondl, M.; and Lau, D. 1979. Social Determinants in Food Selection. *J. Am. Dietet. Assoc.* 74:637.

Richmond, F.W. 1977. The Role of the Federal Government in Nutrition Education. *J. Nutr. Educ.* 9:150.

Schwartz, N.E. 1975. Nutrition Knowledge, Attitudes and Practices of High School Graduates. *J. Am. Dietet. Assoc.* 66:28.

Shapiro, S.S.; Bale, R.L.; and Scardino, V. 1974. *An Evaluation of the Mulligan Stew 4-H Television Series for Extension Service.* Washington, D.C.: U.S. Department of Agriculture.

Shovic, A.M., and Jennings, G. 1979. Effects of Nutrition Education on Nutrition Knowledge, Vegetable Acceptability, and Plate Waste. *School Food Service Res. Rev.* 3:21.

Smith, H., and Justice, C.L. 1979. Effects of Nutrition Programs on Third Grade Students. *J. Nutr. Educ.* 11:92.

Stronck, D.R. 1976. The Need for Nutrition Education. *Am. Biology Teacher* 38:19.

Swanson, J.C. 1972. Second Thoughts on Knowledge and Attitude Effects Upon Behavior. *J. Sch. Health* 42:363.

Talmage, H. et al. 1978. *FOOD . . . Your Choice, Levels 1, 2, and 3 Summative Evaluation.* Technical Report 98. Office of Evaluation Research. Chicago: University of Illinois at Chicago Circle.

Talmage, H.; Hughes, M.; and Eash, M.J. 1978. The Role of Evaluation Research in Nutrition Education. *J. Nutr. Educ.* 10:169.

Talmage, H., and Iverson, B.K. 1979. A Look at School Food Services in Influencing Food Choices: Cases and Instruments. *School Food Service Res. Rev.* 3:65.

Talmage, H., and Rasher, S.P. 1978a. *FOOD . . . Your Choice: A Second Year Follow-up Study.* Technical Report 101. Office of Evaluation Research. Chicago: University of Illinois at Chicago Circle (October).

———. 1978b. *An Initial Exploration of Impact of FOOD . . . Your Choice on Participating School Sites for National Dairy Council.* Technical Report 102. Office of Evaluation Research. Chicago: University of Illinois at Chicago Circle (October).

———. 1980. *FOOD . . . Your Choice Level Four: A Formative Evaluation.* Technical Report 128. Office of Evaluation Research. Chicago: University of Illinois at Chicago Circle.

Terry, R.D.; Bass, M.A.; and Kolasa, K.A. 1979. Rainy Season Food Behavior of Selected East Nicaraguan Miskito Indians. *Home Ec. Res. J.* 8:118.

Todhunter, E.N. 1965. Nutrition Education: Its History, Progress and Problems. Presented as the Mary Swartz Rose Memorial Lecture, New York, April 22.

Tolin, D. et al. 1979. A Comparison of Two Approaches to Nutrition Education at the Third Grade Level. *School Food Service Res. Rev.* 3:24.

Tuckman, B.W. 1979. *Evaluating Instructional Programs.* Boston: Allyn & Bacon.

Ullrich, H.D. 1978. Identifying Needs and Then What? *J. Nutr. Educ.* 10:52.

Wang, M., and Dwyer, J. 1975. Reaching Chinese-American Children with Nutrition Education. *J. Nutr. Educ.* 7:145.

Whitehead, F.E. 1957. Nutrition Education for Children in the U.S. Since 1900. *J. Am. Dietet. Assoc.* 33:(Part I) 880, (Part II) 885.

———. Nutrition Education Research. *World Review of Nutrition and Dietetics* 17:91.

Wishik, S.M., and Van der Vynckt, S. 1976. The Use of Nutritional "Positive Deviants" to Identify Approaches for Modification of Dietary Practices. *Am. J. Pub. Health* 66:38.

Yetley, E.A.D. 1974. A Causal Model Analysis of Food Behavior. Ph.D. thesis, Iowa State University.

Yperman, A.M., and Vermeersch, J.A. 1979. Factors Associated with Children's Food Habits. *J. Nutr. Educ.* 11:72.

3

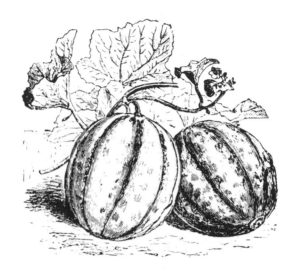

TEACHER TRAINING IN NUTRITION EDUCATION

Joanne P. Nestor

INTRODUCTION

Teacher input through nutrition education classes is only one of many factors influencing children's diets. Nevertheless, the teacher's role is significant because teachers are in a unique position to provide accurate nutrition information and to influence students' food attitudes and behavior. In conjunction with actual food experiences provided by school feeding programs, classroom experiences can have a powerful impact on students. The 1969 White House Conference on Food, Nutrition, and Health (1970) recommended that teachers be trained in the principles of nutrition, but little was done until the passage of PL 95–166 provided funding through the Nutrition Education and Training Program (NETP).

NETP has brought increased awareness of the vital role of school personnel in the nutrition area and has increased the availability of training, but many needs remain vaguely defined or unfilled. Without clearly stated goals and adequate preparation, teachers are severely constrained in their ability to conduct effective nutrition education.

Several states have made some attempts to recognize the need for nutrition education for students by requiring it as part of health education courses or as a separate subject; many have developed their own nutrition education curricula or recommended others for classroom use. But until recently, few states took steps to assure that their teachers could fulfill this demand.

Later chapters addressing nutrition education for children will discuss the finding that programs which increase nutrition knowledge do not necessarily produce desirable changes in nutrition-related behavior. For although a base of valid nutrition information is necessary to make sound food consumption decisions, it is not sufficient: nutrition knowledge is but one of many factors which influence the decisions. This relationship between knowledge and behavior is also true of teachers: training in nutrition does not necessarily render a teacher willing or able to teach nutrition effectively. Thus, although pre- and in-service teacher training in nutrition and nutrition education is needed to produce capable teachers, such training does not guarantee effective nutrition education of children. Byrd-Bredbenner and Greenwood (no date) found no significant correlation between teachers' nutrition knowledge scores and their scores on a test of attitudes toward teaching nutrition.

While this chapter is based upon a review of the nutrition education literature, health education and educational theory per se are beyond the scope of this work. The literature on curricula is reviewed in the reports on the appropriate grade levels; this section is limited to the preservice and in-service training of teachers of grades kindergarten through twelve.

PRESERVICE PREPARATION

In early studies of classroom nutrition education, Bosley (1947) and Semrow (1956) found that teachers were interested in teaching nutrition to their students but felt constrained by their own lack of college-level preparation in nutrition. The situation has improved somewhat today, but lack of teacher preparation is still a major constraint on the implementation of nutrition education programs at all levels (Ferb et al. 1980).

The preservice (college–level) preparation of teachers of all levels rarely includes nutrition. The Education Commission of the States (1975) found that only three states required any coursework in nutrition for the certification of elementary-level teachers, and only one required nutrition for secondary-level certification. But a Nutrition Foundation (1977) survey concluded that no states required nutrition courses for teacher certification. Ferb et al. (1980) found that the NET Program Needs Assessments of twelve states indicated a need for nutrition courses for the certification of high school home economics teachers; five indicated a requirement for health education teachers; and none mentioned a requirement for elementary, science, or "other" teachers.

Table 1 shows the results of several surveys of actual teacher preparation in nutrition, as measured by completion of one or more courses in nutrition (except Cortes, who surveyed "nutrition or health"). Levine (1979) found that, although more home economics teachers had taken nutrition courses, health teachers reached a significantly larger proportion of students and thus had a greater impact. Cook (1977) observed that teachers who had taken nutrition courses were more likely to include nutrition in their curricula, but this association may not be causative. As the table

Table 1
Percent of Teachers Who Have Taken One or More
College–level Nutrition Courses

Study	State	Grade/Subject	Percent
Cortes (1973)	Hawaii	K–3	39.0*
		4–6	15.0*
Cook (1977)	New Jersey and New York	K–6	25.0
Petersen (1972)	Nebraska	Elementary	9.0
			59.0**
Levine (1979)	New Jersey	High school home economics	97.8
		High school health	45.4
		High school science	12.6
Marr (no date)	Pennsylvania	Home economics	98.6
		Health/physical education	62.0
		Life science	37.0
		All 7–12	22.0

*Nutrition or health course.
**College-level course including nutrition (for example, biology, public health).

shows, virtually all the home economics teachers and about half the health education teachers had had nutrition courses; fewer of the other high school teachers and elementary teachers had studied nutrition.

Petersen and Kies (1972) surveyed Nebraska elementary teachers and found that although only 9 percent had taken a separate nutrition course in college, 59 percent had taken other courses (public health, biology, and so forth) which included nutrition education; however, 83 percent had had no instruction in methods of teaching nutrition. A nutrition knowledge test revealed that teachers were not well informed on nutrition, holding many erroneous beliefs regarding fats, sugars, and vitamins. Nevertheless, 63 percent felt that nutrition should be part of the curriculum, 53 percent included nutrition in integrated programs, and 33 percent taught nutrition as a separate unit. Simple correlations showed little relationship between knowledge scores and attitudes. Thus, we cannot assume that increasing teachers' nutrition knowledge will improve their attitudes toward nutrition education. Although the study surveyed classroom teachers, questions relating to nutrition preparation were limited to college courses and did not investigate in-service experience.

Henneman, Fox, and Kreutz (1976) note that home economics teachers in Nebraska frequently teach other subjects as well, although they currently do not extend their nutrition education activities to these other subjects.

No other studies of teacher preservice preparation in nutrition were identified in the literature search. We assume that these results typify teacher preparation and that the measure used (nutrition course) is appropriate. No doubt many of the teachers who have not had a nutrition course nevertheless have had some nutrition training in health, science, or home economics courses. Others rely on television, newspapers, and popular and professional periodicals, which sometimes present outdated or misleading information (Lovett 1970). No studies were identified which related preservice preparation to any classroom nutrition education activities.

IN-SERVICE NUTRITION EDUCATION TRAINING

Appropriate in-service training in nutrition is especially needed not only because of the inadequate preservice preparation described above, but also because advances in nutrition knowledge, curricula, and educational materials necessitate updating even for teachers with some college-level nutrition background.

Furthermore, in-service training may be a more effective way to improve the nutrition education of teachers in general for several reasons. First, declining school populations mean that fewer new teachers will be entering the system, so the focus should be on teachers already in the system (Callahan 1973). Second, many students of education do not become teachers, or they teach in states other than those in which they were educated, so some resources spent on preservice courses are wasted. Finally, in-service courses can be designed more readily or adapted to meet the specific needs of teacher and student (Grogan 1978). The availability of NET Program funds for in-service programs also enhances their feasibility.

The current scope and extent of nutrition education in-service training and its impact on nutrition education in the classroom are not accurately known. The Education Commission of the States (1975) found that two states required in-service nutrition education training for elementary teachers and two for secondary. A survey of New York and New Jersey elementary teachers found that 3.3 percent had attended a foods or nutrition workshop (Cook, Eiler, and Kaminaka 1977). Cortes (1973) found that health or nutrition workshops had been attended by 7 percent of teachers of grades kindergarten through three and 3 percent of teachers of grades four through six; but 52 percent felt that such training was needed. Analysis of the states' Needs Assessments for the NET Program (Ferb et al. 1980) showed that "lack of teacher training opportunities" was seen as a problem by twenty-five states, although teacher workshops were available in every state and were sponsored by thirty-two state departments of education. Specific problems addressed by workshops included teachers' awareness of available curricula and materials (twelve states); access to *reliable* sources of nutrition information (thirteen); curricula overfilled or competency-based (fourteen); and problems of coordination and communication with school food service personnel (thirty-six). In addition, Head (1974) determined that teacher attitudes toward nutrition can influence students' achievement in otherwise controlled circumstances; therefore, workshops must foster positive attitudes toward nutrition education if they are to be effective.

Most in-service programs are developed around specific curricula or materials or are expressly designed to encourage innovative techniques. A few are conducted solely to transfer information about nutrition or about the availability of various materials and curricula. A final category of in-service programs includes those which have been conducted with small groups of teachers as part of academic research in nutrition education. Some of these are discussed here because, while replication of the training might not be practical, there is some information useful to the development of nutrition in-service training.

The literature review also identified a number of studies, or cases, which described in-service programs but did not include any evaluation. Although we cannot know whether such unevaluated exercises were actually fruitful, they are included here for two reasons: (1) they represent a large portion of the available reports, and (2) evaluation techniques development is so rudimentary that often it is difficult to ascertain whether a study was evaluated.

The quality of evaluation of nutrition education is discussed in detail elsewhere in this book; the discussion need not be repeated here except to note that teacher training programs are not an exception to the rudimentary quality of evaluation work which pervades the field.

An additional obstacle to identifying in-service needs and strengths pervades nutrition education: lack of consistency of measures. The evaluation of a teacher in-service program can be based on any of several criteria, but rarely do we find the evaluation carried to the ultimate goal: improvement of students' nutritional status. More often, evaluation is informal or is based on teachers' attainment of short-term training program objectives.

The literature on teacher training programs reveals several factors influencing or describing the programs, any one of which could be used as an organizational basis. For the purpose of this review, programs are reported in the following categories: (1) training in the use of specific curricula, (2) programs primarily functioning to transfer information about nutrition or nutrition education, (3) formal workshops and informal classroom programs which focus on staff development and teachers' needs, and (4) training for home economics teachers.

Curricula-Specific Workshops

Among the leaders in workshop implementation are the National Dairy Council and the Dairy Council Inc. (DCI), formerly the California Dairy Council. Both have developed curricula based on the Basic Four and include teacher training programs as part of the curriculum package.

The DCI program, called Little Ideas at the preschool level and Big Ideas at the elementary level, has reached 4.5 million children since its introduction in 1973 (Niedermeyer 1979), including almost 1 million during 1978–1979 (Zuber and Moerchen 1979). Although the number of teachers trained is not reported, we estimate that if each teacher has twenty-five pupils, the 900,000 children were taught by 36,000 trained teachers. These curricula are discussed further in Chapters Six and Seven.

DCI nutrition consultants conduct two-hour teacher workshops, review basic nutrition information, including the Recommended Daily Allowances for nutrients, and familiarize teachers with the teacher's guide, student materials, and visual aids. Teachers are also briefed on educational methods appropriate for use with the materials, including instructional objectives, and on questions frequently asked by students and their parents (Zuber and Moerchen 1979). Materials are available only to teachers who have attended a brief workshop on their use, and "consumable" pupil materials are replaced annually on request (Niedermeyer 1979). Eighty percent of the teachers reorder the materials (Fisk 1979).

DCI attributes the program's popularity to several factors, which together point to the need for a cohesive approach to classroom education. The Big Ideas program offers to teachers the training, curricula, materials, and support they need, together with evaluation materials and a proven success rate. The program's distribution system is extensive and thorough. However, its main limitation is that it is knowledge-based: all the skills it imparts are abilities to categorize food. Detailed information on individual foods and nutrients is not offered in sufficient detail to enable the student to make decisions outside the Basic Four system. The student confronted with new foods or accustomed to an ethnic diet not discussed in the program often cannot make sound decisions. The question also remains as to whether the students will make wise food choices, given the Big Ideas system. Pilot studies of the program showed small improvements in frequency of eating breakfast or number of Basic Four servings eaten (Zuber and Moerchen 1979, Bell and Lamb 1973, Fisk 1979), but this is not yet a focus of the program. Niedermeyer (1979) states that behavior change is the program's next step. According to one DCI program director, "These basic skills [in the Big Ideas package] can be compared to driving a car. You don't have to know how an internal combustion engine works to operate a car, but you do have to know how to start the engine and fill the tank with gas" (Zuber and Moerchen 1979). What remains is to produce good drivers.

An adaptation of the Big Ideas program was field tested in Canada (Cooper and Philp 1974). Unlike the DCI studies, this program observed a random sample of all teachers who had taken the three-hour in-service session introducing the materials. Over 70 percent of the teachers implemented the program, but most failed to cover all the program objectives at the recommended depth. Teachers from an area in which the school board had strongly endorsed the program covered the objectives more thoroughly. No knowledge gains were found among students of teachers who did not implement the program; the others showed significant gains both in knowledge and in behavior, as measured by the number of food groups included in the day's breakfast. Such an evaluation measure is in keeping with the Canadian program goal of teaching meal balancing but ignores the fact that the Basic Four foods need not necessarily be included in all meals; for example, only two servings from the meat group are recommended daily.

Available since 1977, the National Dairy Council's *FOOD . . . Your Choice* (FYC) is a sequential program also focused on knowledge gains. Many teachers attend two- to six-hour in-service sessions, conducted by local affiliated Dairy Council units. Talmage and Rasher (1978) report that teachers feel they need the training only the first year they use the program; thereafter, most reorder course materials to present in subsequent years (Moncrief 1979).

Many teachers supplement the materials with other articles, but few suggest additions to the FYC curriculum (Talmage and Rasher 1978). A Missouri survey (Moncrief 1979) found that most teachers spend less than half the time estimated for the full program; apparently they are using the materials selectively rather than as intended. Some teachers report difficulty in fitting the activities into an already-filled curriculum. Moncrief suggests that the Dairy Council identify a subset of the most useful activities for implementation in an abbreviated program. Available literature does not describe the teacher-training component but does report that teacher input has been used to modify the initial versions of the program and to assess subjectively the program's effects on students' basic attitudes and behavior (National Dairy Council 1979; Moncrief 1979). A more recent nationwide survey (Brun 1979) of the second year of placement found that the average time allotted had increased and that nearly all trained teachers were using the program. Those who did not use it gave reasons unrelated to the program itself, including not a classroom teacher (nurse, librarian); school policy of teaching nutrition education in alternate years; and team teaching, with another teacher responsible for nutrition education.

Information Transfer Programs

An early experimental in-service program was conducted by the North Carolina State Board of Health. A study of one county's food habits and means of altering them found that the schools' potential contribution was limited by the teachers' inadequate preparation in nutrition and consequent hesitancy to teach it. An eight-hour workshop discussed current knowledge in nutrition and methods and techniques useful at various grade levels (materials are not mentioned). Teachers were also offered individual help in identifying appropriate topics for discussion, based on their own observations and the study findings; sequential lesson guides; and frequent follow-up visits by the staff nutritionist, once the nutrition teaching had begun. The follow-up visit was judged the most valuable service, as it gave teachers added confidence; the program as a whole was judged worthy of replication in other counties. Bosley (1947) points out in the North Carolina study that while teachers are lacking in nutrition knowledge, nutritionists lack education skills, and that collaboration is vital.

Wakefield and Vaden (1973) devised a Telenet program enabling elementary teachers (65 percent of subjects), food service personnel (11 percent), and others (24 percent) to participate in an innovative nutrition education program at branches of Kansas State University. The eight three-hour sessions included presentations on food in the life-style of individuals; digestion, absorption, and utilization of nutrients; physical versus psychological needs for food; and differentiating food facts from fallacies. Teaching objectives, resource materials, lesson plans, and teaching techniques were presented. Wichita Dairy Council staff presented two sessions based on the ubiquitous Big Ideas program. Evaluation consisted of measures of knowledge gain ("significant") and student reports of the degree to which their individual purposes had been met ("moderate"). A limited follow-up study indicated that teachers were actively implementing innovative nutrition programs, but no further description of their activities was sought.

A three-week workshop conducted by the College of William and Mary for fifteen teachers and food service personnel focused on nutrition and physical fitness. Objectives included increasing participants' knowledge of nutrition and its relation to health, how to recognize and deal with nutrition problems, and how to incorporate

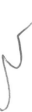

nutrition into the total school program. The group studied nutrition needs from the prenatal period through adolescence, heard speakers, and prepared individual projects incorporating nutrition into their teaching. Response, assessed informally, was enthusiastic but did not lead to innovative ideas. Such standard techniques as tasting parties, visual aids, and food preparation supplemented didactic methods. Success in increasing students' consumption of milk and vegetables in the lunchroom was attributed in part to the course's emphasis on building upon student interests (Parham 1971).

Head (1974) conducted a study of the effects of nutrition education on students at three grade levels. Nine teachers first attended a one-week workshop which included (1) a basic review of nutrition, dietary patterns, and food consumption; (2) a review of publications and visual materials available for students at each level; (3) identification and introduction of resource people from their community; and (4) development of curriculum plans for use during the project. The settings for nutrition education differed greatly among the classes: in the fifth grade classes the program was integrated into several subjects and several activities were conducted; seventh grade nutrition was taught in a health course using conventional teaching methods and tasting parties; and tenth grade students studied nutrition in a biology course which incorporated animal studies and self-assessment of diets. Experiences also varied among teachers. Evaluation based on knowledge, attitude, and behavior changes showed that programs were more successful in classes in which the individual teacher was committed to nutrition. Two teachers known to have "negative feelings about nutrition" used fewer innovative techniques and attained less overall success. Thus, teacher attitudes are shown to be a significant influence on student-based outcomes of training programs.

Staff Development and Teachers' Needs

In discussing the design of local in-service programs, one study notes that ". . . while the consensus among educators is that staff involvement plays a significant role in the success of any inservice program, the fact remains that this practice is more the exception than the rule. In reality, most in-service programs have been planned on the basis of one or two factors: (a) the administrator's personal perceptions of the district's in-service needs; and/or (b) the availability of resources at the local college of education level" (Mangieri and McWilliams 1976, p. 110). A curriculum committee comprised of teachers, staff members, and school administrators reviewed a proposed inservice program for reading and sought feedback from their constituents. The topics were selected through a three-level needs assessment, which included teachers' expressed needs, recommendations of district instructional leaders, and classroom observations conducted by university-level team members. The in-services themselves were competency-based and taught by instructors who had been involved in the needs assessment process and were familiar with participants' strengths and weaknesses. Results showed that participants believed their skills had improved and felt more competent and professional, as evidenced by unprecedented enrollments in graduate courses and professional organizations and interest in professional publications. Students' achievements and attitudes also improved significantly: student gains in reading achievement averaged 1.37 to 1.98 years after only eight months of instruction, and the amount of "free reading" increased. Although the course content of this study was reading rather than nutrition, it does illustrate a useful method for inservice development.

The School Nutrition Education Curriculum Study of Pennsylvania State University conducted a six-week workshop for heterogeneous groups of teachers, food service directors, school nurses, and administrators (Bell 1979). Using a staff development approach, the workshops were intended to inspire participants to incorporate nutrition into their own curricula: the nutrition curriculum itself and the methods for implementation would grow from school needs and resources. A major obstacle was the participants' lack of knowledge about nutrition and bodily functions. There was no agreement as to which activities were appropriate for students at various levels. During the workshop, teachers, when undirected, tended to suggest activities which emphasized food manipulation rather than nutrition understanding. Participants had difficulty designing activities other than health lectures or reading assignments as vehicles for nutrition instruction. These results indicated that teacher workshops alone could not deliver the nutrition education capabilities recommended by the White

House Conference report of 1970. The study group decided to design an instructional program to meet the apparent need for a coordinated, articulated curriculum that exacted higher cognitive thought, skill development, and attention to attitudes toward nutrition that would be more effective in eliciting suitable behavior. Existing materials were seen as projecting values based on acceptance of admonitions and fear of consequences resulting from inattention to nutrition. Such approaches are a common pitfall in dealing with health-related issues, for admonitions and fears are not effective instruments in changing health-related behavior. A major criterion in the subsequent development of the curriculum, "Nutrition in a Changing World," was that "teacher preparation requirements should be as undemanding as possible." At the time of Bell's report, preliminary tests showed significant knowledge gains on the part of students; no further information about teachers was given.

Grogan (1978) asked teachers about their training and curriculum requirements. The teachers were dissatisfied with curricula which neglected their students' real concerns, such as weight control, food supply safety and adequacy, and nutrition for athletes. The few teachers who had some academic background in nutrition desired more up-to-date and topical information. Two in-service courses were designed for teachers of health, home economics, physical education, science, and social studies: one on nutrition information and one on innovative teaching strategies. The courses totaled thirty hours of evening instruction; thirty-five teachers enrolled voluntarily. Based on teacher input, the objectives of the nutrition information course were to (1) develop teacher awareness (and, indirectly, student awareness) of the relevance of nutrition to academic and extracurricular performance; (2) provide information to combat the misinformation of the mass media; and (3) make a variety of reliable nutrition education resources available for classroom use. Thus, teachers were made aware of existing resources and could assess them before taking the in-service training on innovative strategies; most teachers took both courses. Participants made significant gains in nutrition knowledge and expressed an increased sense of competency to teach nutrition.

The second in-service course, Innovative Teaching Strategies, concentrated on a variety of approaches useful in developing comprehensive, interdisciplinary approaches to nutrition education, to counter students' expressed boredom while meeting their actual needs. A resource center and curriculum guide were developed.

Follow-up visits to assess teachers' progress and offer consultation revealed that 70 percent of the teachers were conducting nutrition education programs and that students were exhibiting "much more interest and enthusiasm" than before, although the indicators of this attitude change are not discussed. Student pre- and post-tests did show significant knowledge gains, but three-day food intake records, evaluated using a Basic Four rule for adequacy, showed no diet improvement. Although Grogan admits that this result is in keeping with most other research, she does not consider the possibility that students might have made significant behavior changes overlooked by her dietary evaluation tool. The Basic Four measures servings, not calories; overweight students could have significantly decreased their calorie intakes without affecting their Basic Four profiles. Similarly, reduced consumption of dietary fats (a factor in heart disease) or meat (a response to food supply concerns) might not have been detected.

It is unfortunate that this study's evaluation component did not recognize current issues and student needs as well as had the rest of the program. It should also be noted that participation in the program required extensive time and initiative, and the teachers who volunteered were well motivated before enrolling. Moreover, this study, which enabled each teacher to develop an appropriate curriculum, is as individual and decentralized as possible, in contrast with the widely used Dairy Council programs. Finally, the in-service courses were designed to enable teachers to make the best possible use of existing resources, thus avoiding unnecessary duplication of efforts.

A high school home economics teacher conducted a seven-hour workshop for elementary teachers, and based the program on the following objectives: (1) determine needs to integrate nutrition education into the curriculum; (2) provide nutrition information and promote innovative teaching techniques; and (3) evaluate the degree to which nutrition education techniques were accepted and used (Sodowsky 1973). Although the workshop teacher introduced a variety of existing materials, innovation was encouraged. Participants' responses to a follow-up questionnaire administered at the end of the workshop and again five months later indicated that twenty-three of twenty-five teachers successfully incorporated nutrition education into their classroom activities. Teachers reported increased acceptance of the school lunch, and unsolicited reports from parents indicated that children were encouraging their families to eat better at home. The author lists several methods for improving teacher access to nutrition education resources.

Rhodes (1974) reports anecdotally on a schoolwide nutrition education program initiated by one elementary teacher who had attended a summer nutrition education course; her activities generated enthusiasm among the other teachers. They recruited a local home economics teacher, who offered an extension course on integrating nutrition into the existing curriculum. Enthusiastic teachers reported that school lunch participation improved, plate waste decreased, and children seemed less exhausted after physical education periods, implying that they also were eating better at home.

This project illustrates several significant aspects of nutrition education program success: it relied heavily upon the initiative of one leading individual within the system who recruited administrative support; it addressed teacher and student needs, utilizing feedback mechanisms and minimizing disruption of teachers' existing activities; and it remains virtually unevaluated and unreplicable. Without professional observation, situations such as this will proliferate, and we will not know whether we have lost opportunities to identify and utilize factors contributing to program success or whether unsuccessful programs are perpetuated for lack of appropriate evaluation. Most projects do not even reach the "reportage" stage which this project exhibits. It is possible that extensive and worthwhile teacher training efforts are being conducted and not evaluated or reported. As a valuable asset, the NET Program can help to organize this information if simple and effective systems for evaluating and documenting projects are developed.

Chethik (1974) trained volunteers to work with teachers in the classroom, expecting to train both students and teachers simultaneously, while helping teachers understand and implement an effective nutrition education program. Teachers assisted in the selection and implementation of activities appropriate to the students' age, interests, and achievements. However, difficulties arose, including lack of administrative support, teachers' excessive dependence on the volunteers, and volunteers' demands upon the investigator for "encouragement and support at odd hours." No evaluation was conducted other than acceptance of the method itself: eight of the twenty-two teachers utilized the program the following year.

Parental initiative at a New York City school engendered a singularly successful, though uncontrolled, integrated nutrition education program (Kamhi 1980). Title IV-C funds were used to hire a nutrition consultant to conduct lunch-hour meetings for a small group of teachers. The teachers used a textbook based on food experiences as the basis to develop a program aimed at improving children's intake in comparison to U.S. dietary goals. Sugar, salt, saturated fats, and refined flour gradually were eliminated from the school lunch program as classroom testing experiences introduced children to unrefined grains, meat alternatives, and fruit for snacks and desserts. In response to increasing demands for workshops and recommended foods, NET Program funds were allocated to support the program. All participants considered the program successful.

Programs for Home Economics Teachers

As noted above, home economics teachers are almost universally well prepared in nutrition, if not in nutrition education. Nevertheless, home economics teachers need in-service training to keep up to date with changing nutrition knowledge and education techniques.

Henneman, Fox, and Kreutz (1976) assessed such an update in-service program for twenty teachers. Participants commented after the workshop that the most useful components were the nutrition information update, the opportunity to examine new materials (books, audiovisuals); and laboratory work with food concepts relating to recently developed concerns, such as meatless meals, fat control, and meal management. A questionnaire mailed at the end of the following school year brought a 55 percent response rate, with reports that teachers had replicated many of the laboratory experiences in their own classes, and that they would repeat all the activities of the original workshop. Clearly, the experience and enthusiasm of the teachers contributed to the success of this program. Thus, this study supports the two observations that nutrition education is more effective when food-related activities are used to supplement the more common lecture and discussion techniques, and that sufficiently motivated teachers benefit from increased knowledge of nutrition facts and of new materials.

SUMMARY

Although some states require teachers to study or teach nutrition, most newly graduated teachers are not prepared to conduct nutrition education programs. Fewer than one-third of elementary-level teachers have taken a nutrition course; at the high school level, almost all home economics teachers have studied nutrition, but only about a fifth of all other teachers have taken nutrition courses.

There is no consensus among "nutrition experts" regarding what information students and teachers need, or even how to measure desirable behavior outcomes. Each study and workshop established its own goals and objectives, so although most were successful to some degree, we are not left with a cohesive or logical body of information. Some programs, such as those offered by the Dairy Councils, are capable of delivering a strictly predefined message, while others enable teachers to establish curricula geared to their students' needs. The dilemmas of message content are beyond the scope of this paper, and the evaluation difficulties are discussed in another section. Nevertheless, we can offer several useful observations and conclusions. First, teachers want and need skills in nutrition information and educational methodologies. Second, those skills are best acquired through in-service training rather than preservice, in order to reach the existing pool of teachers and to keep them informed of progress in nutrition information, education techniques, and materials. Third, teachers' attitudes affect students' progress. Finally, despite their discrepancies, the studies identified several features shared by many of the successful programs:

1. Course content and objectives were based on teachers' needs, as they perceived them.
2. Teachers participated voluntarily and were enthusiastic about programs.

3. Teachers became familiar with available resources: materials, curricula, and personnel.
4. Individualized attention was available for meeting unique needs.
5. Nutrition consultants and other specialists provided support services as needed.
6. Courses were attended by other school personnel, including food service managers, nurses, and administrators.

Further work is needed to define both the content and the structure of in-service training. Most studies relied on well-motivated volunteers; we do not have much evidence about what motivated them to participate—we do not know what makes teachers want to teach nutrition. We also lack classroom curricula and materials which teachers can use with confidence to improve students' eating habits. Many states are using NET Program funds to develop innovative teacher inservice programs, but there has not yet been time to design, conduct, evaluate, and report on these courses. As the results of NET Program activities become available, we can look for answers to some of the remaining questions about effective nutrition education training.

BIBLIOGRAPHY

Bell, C., and Lamb, M.W. 1973. Nutrition Education and Dietary Behavior of Fifth Graders. *J. Nutr. Educ.* 5:196.

Bell, P.E. 1979. Adaptation of Nutrition Educator-Determined Objectives for Learner Developmental Levels. Paper presented at the annual meeting of the American Education Research Association, San Francisco, April.

Bosley, B. 1947. A Practical Approach to Nutrition Education for Children. *J. Am. Dietet. Assoc.* 23:304.

Brun, J.K. 1979. *Use of FOOD . . . Your Choice in the Second Year of Placement.* Chicago: National Dairy Council.

Byrd-Bredbenner, C., and Greenwood, B. B. 1979. Nutrition Knowledge and Attitudes of Early Elementary Teachers. Paper presented at the seventieth annual meeting of the American Home Economics Association, St. Louis, June 25–28.

Callahan, D.L. 1973. In-service Teacher Workshops. *J. Nutr. Educ.* 5:233.

Chethik, B.B. 1974. Volunteers Teach Nutrition to Teachers and Students. *J. Nutr. Educ.* 6:133.

Cook, B.; Eiler, D.A.; and Kaminaka, E.C. 1977. How Much Nutrition Education in Grades K–6? *J. Nutr. Educ.* 9:131.

Cooper, B., and Philp, M. 1974. Evaluation of Nutrition Education in Everyday Teaching Environment. *J. Nutr. Educ.* 6:99.

Cortes, M.P., and Standal, B.R. 1973. Nutrition Education Practices in Elementary Schools in Hawaii. *J. Nutr. Educ.* 5:18.

Education Commission of the States. 1975. The Status of Nutrition Education. Denver: Education Commission of the States.

Ferb, T.E. et al. 1980. *The Nutrition Education and Training Program: A Status Report, 1977–1980, Volume I*. Cambridge, Mass.: Abt Associates Inc.

Fisk, D. 1979. A Successful Program for Changing Children's Eating Habits. *Nutrition Today* (May/June): 6.

Grogan, J. 1978. Teacher In-service for Nutrition Education—An Interdisciplinary Approach in the School System. *J. Nutr. Educ.* 10:119.

Head, M.K. 1974. A Nutrition Education Program at Three Grade Levels. *J. Nutr. Educ.* 6:56.

Henneman, A.; Fox, H.; and Kreutz, S. 1976. A Nutrition Workshop for Home Economics Teachers. *J. Nutr. Educ.* 8:25.

Kamhi, M.M. 1980. Making Diets Healthy at P.S. 166. *Nutrition Action* 7:3.

Levine, R.R.; McChesney, A.S.; and Brush, M.K. 1979. An Assessment of High School Nutrition Education. *J. Nutr. Educ.* 11:124.

Lovett, R.; Barker, E.; and Marcus, B. 1970. The Effect of a Nutrition Education Program at the Second Grade Level. *J. Nutr. Educ.* 2:81 (Supplement 1).

Mangieri, J.N., and McWilliams, D.R. 1976. Designing an Effective In-service Program. *J. Teacher Ed.* 27:110.

Marr, T.; Shannon, B.; and Spanier, G. No date. Nutrition Education for Grades 7–12: The Perspective of Teachers and Administrators. Unpublished.

Moncrief, M.H. 1979. An Analysis of *FOOD . . . Your Choice* and Implications for 1978–79 Operations: Results of a Two-Day Planning Workshop Conducted by the St. Louis District Dairy Council. Program Planning Documents for 1978–79 St. Louis District Dairy Council (Executive Summary).

National Dairy Council. 1977. *Food . . . Your Choice: A Nutrition Learning System.* Chicago: National Dairy Council.

Niedermeyer, F.C. 1978. A Comprehensive Study of the Effects and Use of the Dairy Council of California's Two Big Ideas in Nutrition Education Programs for Elementary Schools. Unpublished.

Nutrition Foundation. 1977. Nutrition Education in the Public Schools: An Assessment. Washington, D.C.: Nutrition Foundation.

Parham J.F. 1971. Teacher, There's an Eggplant in the Classroom. *Sch. Lunch J.* 25:62.

Petersen, M.E., and Kies, C. 1972. Nutrition Knowledge and Attitudes of Early Elementary Teachers. *J. Nutr. Educ.* 4:11.

Rhodes, R.J. 1974. Teachers Learn How to Teach Nutrition. *Food and Nutr.* (August): 3.

Semrow, E.N. 1956. The Forward Look in Nutrition Education. *J. Home Econ.* 48:685.

Sodowsky, J.D. 1973. In-Service Nutrition Education for Elementary Teachers. *J. Nutr. Educ.* 5:139.

Talmage, H., and Rasher, S.P. 1978. *Food . . . Your Choice: A Second Year Follow-up Study.* Technical Report 101. Office of Evaluation Research. Chicago: University of Illinois at Chicago Circle (October).

Wakefield, L.M., and Vaden, A.G. 1973. Nutrition Course for Elementary Teachers by Telephone (Telenet). *J. Nutr. Educ.* 5:190.

White House Conference on Food, Nutrition, and Health. 1970. Recommendations of Panels on Nutrition Teaching and Education. *J. Nutr. Educ.* 1:24.

Zuber, S., and Moerchen, B.D. Nutrition Education: It's a Winner! *School Food Service J.* (August): 63.

4

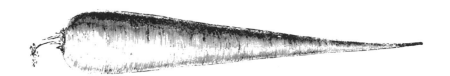

EDUCATION AND TRAINING FOR SCHOOL FOOD SERVICE PERSONNEL

Allene G. Vaden

INTRODUCTION

The introduction of Section 19 of PL 95–166 states: "Congress finds that . . . school food service personnel have not had adequate training in food service management skills and principles, and many . . . school food service operators have not had adequate training in the fundamentals of nutrition" (95th Congress 1977, 91 Stat. 1325). The act authorized implementation of a nutrition information and education program through a system of grants to state educational agencies. Nutritional and food service management training for food service personnel was also included in the act. This chapter examines the background and significant developments in school food service personnel training, the need for training, a description of studies on development and/or evaluation of training materials and programs, and recommendations for school food service training.

With a few exceptions, the review has been limited to publications since 1955, with papers and other publications on school food service training as the primary sources. We also included literature on training related to the general area of food service that had direct applicability to school food service. Four key journals were reviewed: *Journal of the American Dietetic Association, Journal of Home Economics, School Food Service Journal* (formerly, *School Lunch Journal*), and *School Food Service Research Review*. We sought additional post-1955 information from the annual listings of theses and dissertations in home economics, compiled by the Agricultural Research Service (1955–1961) and the American Home Economics Association (1962–1977). Other sources included a selected bibliography on nutrition education and training prepared by Abt Associates Inc. (1979) and the Food and Nutrition Information Center Literature Search on Nutrition Education (1979) prepared for the project. Finally, we reviewed selected publications, proceedings, and other literature, as available.

BACKGROUND AND SIGNIFICANT DEVELOPMENTS
Prior to 1970

According to Flanagan (1971), one of the earliest training programs in school food service was that of the Works Progress Administration (WPA), established in 1935 for the purpose of creating jobs for unemployed adults and youth. Under the WPA, the federal government provided labor and trained supervisory personnel for school lunch programs. WPA guidelines (1940) recommended two to five days of preservice training for project workers, followed by in-service training. District supervisors were to attend preservice and in-service training sessions and, in turn, provide training for county supervisors who would train unit supervisors and workers. WPA manuals dealt with sanitation, space and equipment requirements, food standards, and menu patterns.

Following enactment of the National School Lunch Act in 1946 (PL 79–396), which stimulated rapid growth of the School Lunch Program, the most pressing problem at the local level was obtaining properly trained personnel. Flanagan (1971) indicated that both the state and federal governments attempted to alleviate the situation through workshops and by encouraging high schools and colleges to offer necessary training courses.

Another important development in 1946 was the founding of the American School Food Service Association, which evolved from a merger of the Food Service Directors Conference and the National School Cafeteria Association. One purpose of the new organization was to further the professional growth of its members. Because so few school personnel were trained in quantity food service work, the association placed emphasis on personnel training and improved job performance standards.

Briefly reviewing the initiation of early training programs, Flanagan indicated that most state departments of education were sponsoring or conducting summer school food service training by the late 1940s. Utility company home economists, board of health consultants, and college faculty members provided teaching assistance to state staffs. These summer courses varied from two days to two weeks or more in length and were held in state campgrounds, in schools, and on college campuses. Some training sessions were designed for a single school system or for several systems; however, those held on campuses were generally statewide in scope. Flanagan described several deficiencies of these early training sessions: the wide educational diversity of those attending, from participants with poor reading skills to college graduates, and from food service newcomers to those with extensive experience; the scarcity of qualified instructors; the broad scope of subject matter covered; and limited or nonexistent evaluation and follow-up.

Other significant developments in the early stages of the School Lunch Program related to personnel training and standards were the Southeast regional workshops on school lunch supervision in 1944 and 1945, and the authorization of school lunch certificates for degree personnel in 1947 by the Florida State Board of Education. The certification program was based on qualifications parallel to those for other instructional supervisors.

Garvue, Flanagan, and Castine (1971) report that in 1949, at a national workshop at Iowa State College for state-level food service personnel (cosponsored by the U.S. Department of Agriculture and the U.S. Office of Education, among others), recommendations were developed for education and training programs. These recommendations influenced nationwide practices throughout the 1950s and 1960s.

An early study (*School Feeding in the United States* 1947) indicated that staffing was one of the major national problems of the school lunch program. A sufficient number of trained workers to operate programs effectively, taking into consideration student needs in each school, was cited as a requisite for increasing participation and improving the nutritional adequacy of lunches.

The Southern States Work Conference, initiated in 1940 to examine educational problems, began studying school lunch operations in 1945. The conference proceedings published in 1947 stressed the need for specific training of school lunch personnel (Southern States Work Conference on Educational Problems 1947).

The rapid development of school feeding programs and the pressures to initiate them made it difficult to establish standards for supervisory personnel. In recognition of the need for qualified persons to direct programs, a joint statement was issued in 1948 by the American School Food Service Association, the American Dietetic Association, and the American Home Economics Association on standards for personnel responsible for supervision and management of school lunch programs. The three associations specified educational and experience requirements.

According to Flanagan (1971), many states reported training and personnel developments as achievements of the first decade of the school feeding program. She indicated, however, that although certification standards historically have been used as a means of upgrading personnel in education, as late as 1963 few states had attempted to certify school food service personnel.

The Southern States Work Conference, which continued to work on program policies during the 1950s and 1960s, published a bulletin on school food service standards in 1967 (Flanagan and Martin 1967). Recommended standards concerning state and local staffing and personnel qualifications and training included the following: state certification programs for school food service directors, managers, and personnel; cooperative development of undergraduate and graduate courses by higher education institutions and state education agency and school system-level personnel; and preservice and in-service education for school food service personnel.

Other significant recommendations concerning personnel training needs were made by the second USDA workshop for state school food service directors in 1968, the first such conference since 1946. The Committee on Nutrition Education and Personnel Training recommended that two-year degree programs be established for managers and that four-year degree and graduate programs be established for supervisors. The group also endorsed the 1967 resolution of the National Association of State Universities and Land Grant Colleges (NASULGC) supporting development of more adequate school food service personnel training programs (Flanagan 1971).

Also in response to the NASULGC resolution, the 1968 report of the Joint Committee on Education for Government Service (of USDA and land grant universities) indicated that a school lunch task force had been appointed "to study mechanisms to encourage, evaluate, coordinate and fund research and training programs for school food service personnel at federal, state and local levels." The task force, after reviewing data from several surveys, found that the need for training and education was continuous and existed at all levels, but was most critical at the worker or unit manager level. While most states were concerned about training, the task force concluded that without objective evaluation of training, the effectiveness of training efforts would remain unclear (Garvue, Flanagan, and Castine 1971).

The task force's recommended plan of action included regional seminars for school food service professionals, regional centers and traineeships for graduate study, expansion of vocational and community college training programs for unit managers and workers, and establishment of an education materials center. A prototype seminar on management functions was held at the University of Tennessee in the summer of 1969 and was followed by three additional regional seminars in 1970 also on management functions (University of Tennessee 1969; U.S. Department of Agriculture, Food and Nutrition Service 1971).

The 1970s

PL 91–248, enacted in 1970, allowed use of up to 1 percent of child nutrition program funds for nutritional training of workers, coordinators, and participants of the programs, as well as for surveys and studies of requirements for food service programs; permitted states to use up to 1 percent of apportioned funds for special developmental projects; and established a National Advisory Council on Child Nutrition (PL 91–248, 91st Congress 1970; Gunderson 1971). These provisions were significant, because funds were made available for strengthening training, research, and development efforts, which many authorities had been promoting since the early days of the program. Garvue, Flanagan, and Castine (1971) contended that the lack of funds had handicapped program development.

Another significant development was completion in 1971 of the two-year National School Food Service and Nutrition Education Finance Project, one of eleven satellite studies of the National Educational Finance Project. A key conclusion of the study stressed that effective school nutrition programs are contingent on continuous efforts to increase personnel effectiveness. The study emphasized the importance of preservice and in-service education programs to train personnel in appropriate skills as food service technology and program policies change. The study also emphasized the need to determine training program effectiveness and to explore cooperative training within the entire food service industry as a means of using resources effectively and avoiding duplication of efforts (Garvue et al. 1971).

Five regional seminars were held in the summer of 1971 with funds from PL 91–248 (Pennsylvania State University 1971, Florida Agricultural and Mechanical University 1971, University of Wisconsin–Madison and Extension 1971, Kansas State University 1971, Utah State University 1971). The seminars provided academic training and education for supervisory personnel in the expanded role of school food service in nutrition education (U.S. Department of Agriculture, Food and Nutrition Service 1971). Other training and development efforts also were funded, including materials development and television training programs, and a five–state project involving a team approach to training food service personnel and teachers (Georgia Department of Education 1975, Luck 1979). We will look at the design and evaluation of the seminars and project in the section on programs.

The National Advisory Council on Child Nutrition, begun in 1971, became active in reviewing and making recommendations on all aspects of the programs, including personnel training (National Advisory Council on Child Nutrition 1972–1976, 1979). Findings and recommendations related to training programs are summarized in a subsequent section of this paper.

The American School Food Service Association, begun in 1946, has been another important force in human resource development in school food service. The association has always promoted the professional growth of its members through publications, workshops, and meetings. Efforts were expanded in the 1970s with development and reorganization of a certification program, specification of competency statements, and redirection of association committees on education and training.

TRAINING NEEDS

Need in the job context has been described as a lack of knowledge, skill, or attitude that prevents an employee from performing satisfactorily or that interferes with his or her potential for assuming greater responsibilities (Hospital Continuing Education Project 1970).

Needs assessment is specified in the legislation as a requisite of the NET Program and is delineated with more specificity in the regulations (PL 95–166, 95th Congress 1977; U.S. Department of Agriculture, Food and Nutrition Service 1979). The literature has emphasized repeatedly the importance of needs assessments in the design of education and training programs (Claycombe, Bird, and Bennett 1976; Hospital Continuing Education Project 1970; Lester 1973; Newell 1976).

In this section, we review the recommendations of the National Advisory Council on Child Nutrition and national studies on personnel training needs; we also summarize studies reported since 1955 that were designed as needs assessments.

Recommendations of the National Advisory Council

The first five annual reports of the National Advisory Council on Child Nutrition included recommendations on upgrading school food service personnel (1972–1976, 1979). The first report recommended that the U.S. Department of Agriculture provide leadership and coordination with the state departments of education and professional groups to upgrade personnel; this would be accomplished by developing staffing patterns and qualifications for food service personnel and by further encouraging community colleges, universities, and other institutions to provide training. Several specific actions were recommended:

1. The competencies required for food service work should be determined.
2. Standards and qualifications for personnel involved in food service work should be established.
3. Curriculum for both preservice and in-service training of school food service personnel should be developed.
4. Funds for training school food service personnel should be identified and used, with particular attention to state and federal funds available for vocational educational and manpower training.
5. Manuals on school food service operations should be available in all programs. (National Advisory Council on Child Nutrition 1972)

The council's 1973 annual report noted the need for federal

emphasis on training trainers. Educating trainers in nutritional science, nutrition education, and food service management operations was underlined as a priority for federal funds. The report stressed that trained food service personnel would be a valuable resource for nutrition education.

The following year's report (1974) recommended continued efforts to upgrade personnel as essential to improving programs and increasing participation. The fourth annual report (1975) emphasized the need for adequate numbers of appropriately trained state staff to assist state departments of education in monitoring and advising local programs. The council reviewed progress on training projects authorized by PL 91–248 in these two reports (1974, 1975) and in the fifth report (1976). Also during 1975, the council concentrated on recommendations to strengthen nutrition education, including emphasis on team approaches which encourage cooperation between teachers and school food service personnel (1976). The 1977 report included a review of progress on training (1979), but no recommendations.

National Studies

Although not directed at training needs, the 1971–1972 study by the U.S. Department of Agriculture of high school participation in school lunch suggested the need for employee training. Negative attitudes, lack of understanding of program goals, and failure to merchandize the school lunch were aspects of program operations found in schools with low rates of participation (U.S. Department of Education, Food and Nutrition Service 1978). A random sample of 2,300 public and private schools represented schools in all states (except Hawaii) and included those with small (fewer than 500 students) and large enrollments; results were tabulated from questionnaires administered to 1,126 managers and 7,386 other personnel. Particular emphasis was placed on education, experience, training completed, and training desired, and training was examined in detail. More than six out of ten food service managers were promoted or hired as managers without prior training. Several other findings are pertinent:

 Most available courses were provided by state and local school districts (30 percent and 28 percent, respectively).

Approximately one-half (50.2 percent) reported that training was required.

Approximately 75 percent of the skilled and semiskilled workers reported that training was required.

Approximately 75 percent of those participating reported that on-the-job training was required (as opposed to training courses).

The top five subject areas in which training has been received in the last five years are sanitation/kitchen safety, use and care of equipment, quantity food preparation, nutrition, and menu planning.

No apparent differences in the type of courses in which training had been received were noticed when examined across skill level groupings, grade groupings, or geographic locations.

Only three out of ten food service employees completed training in the past ten years.

The most recent training occurred prior to 1975.

The most common reason for training was the desire to improve job performance.

There was no consensus as to why employees had not been trained.

Analysis of the respondents' desire for more training revealed the following:

Forty-four percent indicated a desire for more training.

The most desired courses were "Nutrition," "Quantity Food Preparation," and "Menu Planning."

Interest in more training increased with years of service up to the tenth year, then dropped off significantly.

Summer was the overwhelming choice as a time for more training, rather than afternoons or evenings during the school year.

The principal reasons for wanting more training were to improve job performance, increase knowledge, and learn new techniques. Suggestions for improving training courses attended included easier access to training site, greater frequency of classes, better course quality, and more subject variety.

Among the recommendations offered to the U.S. Department of Agriculture were the following:

1. Evaluate the feasibility of establishing a career development program for food service workers.

2. Recommend to local school districts that formal training become a prerequisite for advancement.
3. Provide guidance to state agencies for developing materials for training courses.
4. Encourage the development of college training programs for school food service workers.
5. Develop a close working relationship with the states in developing a training course sponsor appraisal program.
6. Work with state and local school districts to make training more accessible to food service workers.
7. Offer courses during working hours with pay and subsidize costs of courses and transportation.

Other Studies

Needs identification studies, in particular methodology and results, are presented here in chronological order.

Fisher (1955) used an industrial technique to provide school lunchroom managers the opportunity to identify improvement needs prior to constructing a training program. By means of job analysis, job evaluation, and a questionnaire, the improvement needs of twenty-three nonprofessional public school lunchroom managers in Dearborn, Michigan, were identified.

In the job analysis section, the duties and responsibilities of the lunchroom managers were defined and classified into job factors, attributes, and subattributes which make job evaluation possible. The author prepared descriptions for each of the three subdivisions of lunchroom manager.

A job evaluation committee determined the relative worth of the job factors, attributes, and subattributes in the overall job of the lunchroom manager. The degree to which each attribute and subattribute entered into the three levels of the job was established.

A questionnaire, with statements suggested by the attributes and subattributes, was prepared for distribution to each lunchroom manager in the survey group. Based on an analysis of the questionnaire, the curriculum for a short- and long-term training program for lunchroom managers was developed. The program was designed so that training would relate to improvement need.

The curriculum of the short-term training program was developed from the statement score of the questionnaire items ranked in order of importance; in the curriculum of the long-range program, both the number and the sequence of the training sessions were determined by the extent to which training would be of value to lunchroom managers. The discussion topics pertained to specific areas that lunchroom managers had noted on their questionnaire as being most valuable in performing their supervisory job.

The value of this study is twofold: it outlines a procedure for identifying the improvement needs of a supervisory group, and it explains the development of a training program that responds to these needs.

Riggs (1956), using a mail survey, studied training in quantity food production offered at the secondary school level in programs in nine midwestern states. Using criteria formulated for the study, the programs were evaluated, and recommendations formulated. Nine criteria for program evaluation were advanced.

Childers (1961) interviewed a sample of lunchroom managers and school administrators to explore the need for competent supervision of local programs in Mississippi. The following questions guided the research:

1. Do the managers of local school lunch programs have the education and training to assume the responsibilities of the work?
2. What responsibilities for the school lunch program are managers assuming?
3. What are the problems of the managers in operating school lunch programs?
4. What commodities are received in the schools, and how valuable are they in the operation of the program?
5. What responsibilities do school administrators assume for the school lunch program?
6. Do administrators desire competent supervision for local school lunch programs?

One Mississippi county was singled out as an example of a consolidated district. Problems in operating the lunchroom reflected the need for competent supervision. All school administrators assumed some responsibility in the operation of the school lunch program. When the administrators listed their assumed managerial tasks, all were in the province of a person normally employed for program supervision. Twelve of the thirteen administrators interviewed favored employing a supervisor and stated that in-service training of employees was one of the greatest problems.

Using data from questionnaires distributed to all school superintendents and school lunch directors in the state of Washington, Helber (1964) identified the essential qualifications and feasibility of establishing a program of certification for school lunch directors. Several needs were identified, including planning kitchen layouts and purchasing for daily operation. Directors indicated a need for further study in other areas: nutrition, personnel management, care of equipment, and business procedures in that order. Superintendents cited personnel management and business procedures as two areas for study. The majority of school superintendents preferred to employ college graduates; the larger school districts required college graduates, indicating that a Master's degree was desirable but not required.

School lunch directors indicated they spent the major portion of their time on business and financial procedures, menu planning, and purchasing for daily operation. The school superintendents indicated that school lunch directors should or would spend a larger portion of their time on personnel management, menu planning, and business and financial procedures.

School lunch directors considered themselves most competent in the areas of purchasing for daily operation, business procedures, menu planning, and personnel management, in that order. The school superintendents considered school lunch directors most competent, first, in menu planning and, second, in purchasing food for daily operation.

Almost two-thirds of the school lunch directors indicated a program of school lunch certification for future school lunch directors should be developed. When asked, "Do you feel that a special certificate should be developed to adequately qualify future school lunch directors?" fewer than a third of the school superintendents answered in the affirmative. School lunch directors desired to upgrade their profession by establishing qualifications for successful school food management. They believed that a qualified director could better promote the business aspect as well as the importance of health and well-being of growing schoolchildren.

In companion studies, Clarke (1966) and Gunn (1966) investigated the knowledge, attitudes, and managerial abilities of Mississippi school lunch managers. Clarke constructed an interview guide with twelve categories considered essential to performance of the school lunch manager's job: controlling sanitation; controlling production standards; maintaining standards of serving; overseeing nutrition in meals; planning, ordering, and purchasing food; maintaining the use of commodities; keeping necessary records and financial controls; establishing duties and scheduling work for all employees; supervising and assisting employees; supervising and assisting in food preparation and service; conducting educational programs for workers; and instructing employees regarding policies and practices.

Clarke chose school lunch managers of eighteen schools within a ninety-mile radius of Hattiesburg, Mississippi. The schools had enrollments of 400 and over. The managers received the lowest rating in records and financial controls, indicating a possible weakness in their educational programs. Overall, the Mississippi managers were well-prepared in such areas as use of commodities, control of sanitation, preparation of food, employee supervision, scheduling of work for employees, and standards of serving. The managers were rated lower than expected in the area of maintaining nutrition in meals. What seemed to be lacking was the more technical managerial knowledge needed to perform efficiently.

Gunn (1966) focused on identification of attitudes related to competency, and development and evaluation of an attitude measurement scale. The initial scale was evaluated by a panel, and the revised scale was completed by a selected sample of school lunch managers. While Gunn urged further work to validate the scale, she also suggested use of the scale for assessing the effects of training programs.

Boudreaux (1972) was concerned with the minimum standards of academic preparation and experience for school food service supervisory personnel, as recommended by food service directors, school food service supervisors, and college personnel in related areas. The five-section survey questionnaire was compiled using recommendations of the Southern States Work Conference, sample certification requirements prepared by the joint committee of representatives from the Association of School Business Officials and the American School Food Service Association, and the catalogs of selected universities. The importance of a baccalaureate degree was the topic of the first section; the next three sections contained a detailed list of courses; and the last section concerned the value of experience with supporting items.

The study revealed that a majority of respondents thought that school food service supervisory personnel should hold a baccalaureate degree as a minimum standard. Recommended courses were classified as core, science/food science, and related areas. The majority indicated that experience be included in the minimum standards, with the four types of experience listed in the questionnaire (trainee, manager, related areas, and laboratory experience in food service at the college level) shown as acceptable. The following recommendations were drawn from the study findings:

1. A certification program for school food service supervisory personnel should be established.
2. Guidelines of minimum standards for school food service supervisory personnel should be established. These guidelines would be used by employment agencies and groups establishing certification requirements.
3. Further study is needed to determine the number of hours of course work needed to meet minimum standards for school food service supervisory personnel.

With the exception of the Boudreaux study, none of the studies focused on program and training needs in school food service. Several of the papers reviewed in the subsequent section on descriptions of training programs included determination of need as a basis for planning.

One of the first studies of the NET Program, reported by Kende et al. (1980), concerned nutrition education and training needs of Michigan school food service directors and supervisors. The survey was designed to collect baseline data on the characteristics of the food service directors and supervisors, the nutrition education programs they currently offer their staffs, and their own need for and interest in additional education and training in nutrition education. Key findings of the research included the following:

Most respondents did not provide nutrition education for their staffs; a few reported receiving some assistance in this effort from other organizations (for example, Dairy Council, Extension).

Respondents indicated that nutrition education could be included in staff meetings and that lesson plans would aid these efforts.

Respondents reported limited involvement in nutrition education for school children.

Except in the area of payroll, about two–thirds of the respondents indicated either a moderate or great need for additional
training in seventeen topical areas surveyed, including topics
in management and nutrition education.

Seventy-eight percent or more were interested or very interested
in additional training in a broad range of topics, such as nutrition, nutrition education, food science, food production and
service, and program merchandizing.

Most preferred regional one-day workshops.

Based on the study results, Kende et al. developed training program recommendations for school food service directors and supervisors in Michigan. They recommended that workshops on topics
of greatest interest to directors and supervisors be the initial
thrust, that directors and supervisors already involved in nutrition
education be enlisted to assist in training others, and that seminars
on the goals of nutrition education be offered.

Related Literature

A few studies were identified which have implications for food
service personnel training. Several studies were concerned with
the effect of training on labor turnover. Gibson and Scoular (1962)
and Pelto and Sweatt (1965) studied food service personnel turnover and concluded that well-defined induction and training programs were effective in promoting job satisfaction and stability.

Using two school districts in the state of Washington, Yaussy
(1970) studied the effect of a required pre-employment training
course on turnover rate. Data from the study were inconclusive,
although some evidence supporting the value of the training was
found among the more skilled classifications of employees.

The fourth study (Harwood and Brown 1968), in the field of
hospital food service, is included here because of its possible general application to other segments of institutional food service, including school food service. The researchers studied the type,
composition, and intensity of preservice and in-service training of
hospital food service workers, and the relationship of such training
to labor turnover and job satisfaction. Data collected in twenty

hospitals in the Baltimore-Washington area led to findings much more clear-cut than those of Yaussy. Hospital food service departments that offered the most concentrated indoctrination, orientation, and training programs had the lowest rates of avoidable turnover. There appeared to be a positive relationship between quality of training programs and job satisfaction, although data in this area were inconclusive.

Hopkins, Vaden, and Vaden (1979) studied school food service employees in twenty-four midwestern schools, documenting the positive relationship between job performance and job satisfaction; that is, school food service employees who reported greater job satisfaction had higher supervisory performance ratings than did those who were less satisfied. Also, the researchers found that food service workers with higher performance ratings had longer tenure in their schools. A second paper from the Hopkins study (1980) documented positive relationships among job performance, job satisfaction, and identification with the organization.

Data from these studies have implications for training needs and the value of training. Reviewed in total, relationships among turnover, training, job performance, and job satisfaction, as reflected in these studies, indicate that training can ease the organizational and quality problems attributed to high rates of turnover.

One other aspect of the research reported by Hopkins, Vaden, and Vaden (1980) deserves mention because of a suggested training need. In an evaluation of the importance of various school food service goals, the authors reported that school food service personnel rated student involvement in the program as the least important goal. In view of federal regulations issued in response to PL 94–105 (U.S. Department of Agriculture, Food and Nutrition Service 1979; PL 94–105 1975), requiring student involvement, the authors expressed concern about this finding. The implication is that food service personnel should receive training that emphasizes the value of, and need for, student involvement.

As defined above, need in the job context describes a lack in knowledge, skill, or attitude that interferes with satisfactory performance. Garrett and Vaden (1978) found a direct relationship between student attitudes and perceptions of food service employees' attitudes. Students' attitudes toward the food and the program were negatively influenced when personnel were viewed as "often crabby."

TRAINING MATERIALS AND PROGRAMS

Literature on school food service personnel training materials and programs is limited to reports in the key professional journals and is categorized as follows: reports on training efforts at the federal, state, and local school district levels; the education and training efforts of the American School Food Service Association (ASFSA), with particular emphasis on the certification program and the competency development project; and university research on training materials and programs. These five categories overlap, however, because of joint sponsorship and planning of programs. For example, the section on federal programs includes several reports of federally funded projects at the state level that appeared to be intended as training models for implementation in other areas.

Discussion of federal training efforts is centered on the 1967 report of the School Lunch Task Force (University of Tennessee 1969). Few state and district training programs were reported in the periodical literature. Although we recognize that most state agencies and local school districts sponsor ongoing summer training programs, conduct or fund other types of training during the school year, and often publish and disseminate extensive training materials for use throughout their states, accounts of these efforts are not readily available.

Several of the university research projects were sponsored cooperatively by colleges or universities and state agencies. These studies are discussed in the research section, not under state training, since the reports were under the aegis of the respective universities.

U.S. Department of Agriculture
Training Efforts

Major impetus for increased federal involvement came in the late 1960s and early 1970s. First, the School Lunch Task Force, authorized by the Joint Committee of the U.S. Department of Agriculture (USDA) and NASULGC on Education for Government Service, formulated several recommendations that had an impact on USDA training and related efforts. The next major force was the enactment of PL 91–248 with its provisions for funding of training, studies of program operations, and developmental projects.

The tremendous expansion of the child nutrition programs in the late 1960s, an outgrowth of public concern regarding the extent of poverty and nutritional problems among the U.S. population (Flanagan 1971, Martin 1978), created many new jobs in school food service and a concomitant need for training.

The seminars sponsored by USDA in 1969 and 1970 were held in response to recommendations of the task force (Goertz 1969; U.S. Department of Agriculture, Food and Nutrition Service 1971). The 1971 USDA regional seminars were among the first training projects funded under authorizations of PL 91–248.

The prototype seminar, held in 1969 at the University of Tennessee, was entitled "Management Functions for State and System Level School and Nonschool Food Service Administrators." It had two objectives: (1) develop an understanding of management functions and their application to the school food services field, and (2) develop materials for use in future food service seminars (Goertz 1979). The schedule for the two-week seminar included daily formal presentations, followed by group discussions. Approximately one hundred districts and state-level personnel attended, primarily from states in the USDA Southeast Region. Participants developed plans for proposed regional, state, and local seminars. The purpose of the seminar planning project was to stimulate a "multiplier" effect, by which training would be extended to other school food service administrators. Graduate credit was available for those interested. An appointed evaluator and ombudsman assisted in identifying feasible changes during the progress of the seminar and was responsible for the overall evaluation report to USDA.

The three USDA regional seminars held in 1970 also focused on management functions; proceedings from two of the seminars were available for review. The emphasis of the Southeast Region Seminar was on the application of management functions to centralized food service systems, and its purposes were: "(1) to improve the management functions of centralized food services for school and day care centers for more effective child nutrition programs and (2) to discuss and define the transitional operation needed to convert a decentralized food service unit to a centralized system" (University of Tennessee 1970). The format was similar to the 1969 seminar, with formal presentations followed by group work sessions each day during the two-week session. Participants developed "plans for action" in which ideas presented during the seminar were incorporated into written procedures for centralizing a portion of their respective food service systems. Plans were reviewed by staff from each district director's state.

The Southwest Region Seminar, "New Concepts in Management," was attended by approximately one hundred state staff and district directors, primarily from the USDA Southwest Region (Oklahoma State University 1970). Its purposes were "(1) to stimulate utilization of group dynamics and (2) to develop the dimensions of management" (Oklahoma State University 1970). The format was similar to that of the Southeast Region Seminar, with presentations and group work. During the seminar, participants wrote plans for projects (involving some management situations), which were to be completed as part of their job at home. Final reports were due to the participants' respective state directors within six months after the seminar.

The 1971 seminars were held at land grant universities in each of the five USDA/FNS regions which existed at that time* (Pennsylvania State University, Florida Agricultural and Mechanical University, University of Wisconsin-Madison and Extension, Kansas State University, and Utah State University). Funded by moneys made available by PL 91–248, the seminars all emphasized nutrition education and related processes in response to provisions of the legislation which authorized nutrition training and education.

Following guidelines established by USDA (1971), seminar objectives and programs were planned within each region by committees, which included representatives from USDA, state agencies, and sponsoring universities. All the seminars were two weeks, and funding was provided for one hundred school food service district directors and state agency personnel. The USDA/FNS established selection criteria and state quotas.

Goals and objectives for the five seminars are listed in Table 1. The primary instructional strategies were formal presentations, panel discussions, case study analyses, reading assignments, and group projects and discussions. Seminar projects were required by all except the Western Region Seminar.

---

*States are currently divided into seven regions.

Table 1
USDA Regional Seminars, 1971—Topics and Objectives

Region/Topic/University	Goal(s)/Objectives
NORTHEAST REGION Topic: "Nutrition Education: Nutrition Delivery Systems and the Management Function" Pennsylvania State University	*Overall objective:* To provide participants with information, resources, and techniques to conduct nutrition education workshops and/or training. *Subgoals:* 1. To review basic food and nutrition concepts and current research. 2. To explicate the interface of the school food service supervisor's significant publics.
SOUTHEAST REGION Topic: "Materials and Methods in Nutrition Education" Florida Agricultural and Mechanical University	*Objectives:* 1. Improvement in supervisory functions in the changing scene of nutritional care. 2. Expansion of knowledge of public programs supportive to nutrition education. 3. Motivation for follow-up nutrition education activities in respective locales. 4. Improvement of skills in developing materials relevant to nutrition education. 5. Increased familiarity with available resources and implementation procedures. 6. Basic planning for nutrition education integration with school food service as an educative tool in the process.
MIDWEST REGION Topic: "Nutrition Education and Related Management Processes" University of Wisconsin, Madison	*Goal:* To provide the impetus and stimulus needed to develop and strengthen leadership abilities of supervisory personnel in school food service, enabling them to contribute toward and participate in child nutrition education programs.

Table 1 (cont.)

Region/Topic/University	Goal(s)/Objectives
SOUTHWEST REGION *Topic:* "Innovative Approaches to Nutrition Education and Related Management Processes" Kansas State University	*Objectives:* 1. To create an awareness of current trends and a desire for further knowledge in nutrition among school food service supervisory personnel. 2. To stimulate an interest in effective techniques that will cause behavioral changes in the nutrition of children. 3. To utilize innovative instructional tools, methods, and media for effective school nutrition programs. 4. To make supervisors aware of the potential value and the necessity of training school food service personnel in nutrition education. 5. To encourage coordination between ongoing education processes in the classroom and the Child Nutrition Programs.
WESTERN REGION *Topic:* "Nutrition Education in the School Food Service—Challenge, Change and Commitment" Utah State University	*Objectives:* 1. To update supervisory personnel in nutritional trends and knowledge so that they more effectively carry the message of nutrition to the local level of school food service. 2. To develop a better understanding of the interrelationship of economic, cultural, social and physical factors which directly affect nutrition problems and nutrition education programs. 3. To develop innovative instructional tools, methods and materials which may be used efficiently and effectively in developing realistic child nutrition programs. 4. To make food service supervisory personnel aware of the necessity for

cooperating with other school personnel, such as superintendents, for help
in implementing their nutrition education programs.

Sources: Penn State University, Florida Agricultural and Mechanical University, University of Wisconsin–Madison and Extension, Kansas State University,
Utah State University

Table 2
USDA Midwest Region Seminar Evaluation

Measure	Session Content	Session Process
Effectiveness	Posttest grade 25% Final project grade 75%	Daily participant evaluation (sample) State group evaluation Session check list
Appropriateness	Daily participant evaluation (sample) State group evaluation	Daily participant evaluation (sample) State group evaluation Session check list
Utility	Self-Evaluation Before, immediately after, three months after, six months after	

Source: University of Wisconsin–Madison and Extension.

A committee with a USDA representative not only planned but
also evaluated each seminar. In addition, the sponsoring university
had designed an evaluation plan. The evaluation schema varied
greatly among the seminars, from emphasis only on evaluation of
the seminar sessions to comprehensive cognitive, affective, and
action domain evaluations. Overall, the evaluation summaries of
USDA were positive, indicating that the objectives of the various
seminars had been met (U.S. Department of Agriculture, Food and
Nutrition Service 1976).

In the Northeast Region Seminar, specified criteria for graduate
or undergraduate credit required completion of a written project
(Pennsylvania State University 1971).

In the Southeast Region Seminar, participants evaluated formal sessions daily as to perceived contribution to their professional growth and knowledge; seminar activities were rated on a three-point scale as excellent, satisfactory, or inadequate. Overall, ratings were quite positive (Florida Agricultural and Mechanical University 1971).

The evaluations of the Midwest and Southwest Region Seminars were the most extensive. As seen in Table 2, effectiveness, appropriateness, and utility were the measures for evaluation in the Midwest; data were collected daily during and periodically after the seminar (University of Wisconsin–Madison and Extension 1971).

To measure the *effectiveness* of the session process and content, a sample of participants evaluated the sessions daily, each of the eleven state groups prepared a composite evaluation, and a seminar faculty member prepared a session check list for reference when analyzing data from other evaluations.

In addition, each day a random sample of thirty participants rated the topics and sessions on that day's schedule, using criteria for content and process *appropriateness.* Participants evaluated the discussion groups, lectures, and panel discussions on the following dimensions: use of interesting techniques, suitable combination of techniques, and effectiveness in achieving learning. "Above average" for all items but one was the evaluation of 50 percent or more of the participants.

To rate seminar *utility,* half the participants completed the series of self-evaluations at four different times: before, immediately after, three months after, and six months after the seminar. Usefulness was indicated by the increased use of community resources which support school food service program activities.

In the Southwest Region Seminar, cognitive and affective learning, as well as innovative efforts following the seminar, were the criteria for assessing effectiveness (Vaden 1973). The objectives of the evaluation were (1) to measure participants' cognitive learning of nutrition and related topics; (2) to measure attitudinal change related to descriptions of organizational role and to receptivity and flexibility ratings; (3) to study relationships among innovation efforts and two methods of continuing contact following the seminar (periodic group conferences and periodic telephone contacts); (4) to study personal and organizational factors related to cognitive learning, attitude change, and innovation efforts; and (5) to study interrelationships among cognitive learning, attitude change, and innovation efforts.

The evaluation plan included two phases: the first, evaluation of cognitive and affective learning, occurred right after the seminar, and the second, evaluation of innovative efforts in the work setting, occurred during the nine months following the seminar.

Two sets of pre- and post-tests were administered: cognitive tests to measure the learning of nutrition and related topics, and attitude scales to assess changes in description of organizational role (measured by shifts in importance and time ratings of position elements) and to measure changes in receptivity and flexibility.

Program speakers submitted items for the cognitive tests. Alternate forms of the test were used because of the short period between pre- and post-test administrations. Items were matched for content and divided between the pre- and post-tests. True/false and multiple choice items were used to insure objective scoring of tests. Each test consisted of thirty-six items related to nutrition education and twenty-two items related to other topics. An overall test score, two subpart scores, and an information gain were derived for statistical analysis.

As part of the attitudinal testing, a fourteen-element instrument was developed to measure shifts in description of organizational role in nutrition education. The instrument consisted of seven nutrition-related and seven administration-related position elements. These elements represented the types of activities in which school food service personnel might be involved and were not intended to provide all-inclusive descriptions. Importance and time ratings were developed as a basis for assessment of relative and absolute changes in position descriptions. The pretest instrument asked for a description of present position in relation to the two rating scales (time and importance) and the fourteen position elements; the post-test asked for a description of planned position for the next school year. In addition, pre- and post-descriptions of an ideal position were included to provide perceptions of organizational role devoid of environmental constraints. Importance and time ratings were weighted one (minor importance or small time allotment) to four (very important or large time allotment). Three scores were derived from each of the four scales: a nutrition activity score, an administrative activity score, and a relative importance of nutrition activity score; two change scores were derived.

A twelve-item scale was developed to measure receptivity or openness to new ideas. Several items concerned willingness to implement innovative ideas, while others implied a degree of social interaction. The items, which included both positive and negative statements, were rated according to a five-point scale (strongly disagree to strongly agree). A twenty-two-item flexibility scale was adapted from that of the California Psychological Inventory (Rutgers University, and Food and Nutrition Services 1972). The scale measured degree of attitude rigidity, and the true/false response was expanded to a five-point rating, from definitely false to definitely true.

The criteria for evaluation of innovation efforts included completion of a project related to seminar objectives, project quality, and extent of nutrition education–related activities during the academic year following the seminar. The participants were subdivided into three experimental groups to assess the influence of postseminar contact on innovation efforts:

Group I: Group conferences (meeting group). Consultants from the seminar met with Group I three times to determine application of results of seminar and progress on individual projects in nutrition education and to plan for adaptations.

Group II: Telephone contact (phone group). Long-distance telephone calls were made to each of the seminar participants by a consultant at regular intervals to check on changes made on the basis of seminar content and to encourage the implementation of innovative ideas.

Group III: No contact (control group). Participants returned to home station without formal or planned contacts until the regional follow-up of the entire group at the end of the school year.

The study sample was stratified by state, position, and type of project proposed, then randomly assigned to contact groups.

Project ideas submitted to seminar faculty at the end of the first week were reviewed and returned with suggestions for preparation of a tentative outline, which was filed prior to the end of the seminar. Each outline was evaluated for completeness, clarity, and apparent feasibility within the organizational setting described. It was returned with an attached memorandum enumerating specific suggestions for implementation of the project and guidelines for preparation and submission of the final project outline. This correspondence was timed to reach the study sample shortly after the academic year began. A three-member panel evaluated projects on degree of relevance to nutrition education, extent of apparent impact on target group, and resourcefulness of the project director in designing the project.

A survey instrument, based on seminar objectives, was distributed at the end of the academic year to all seminar participants; its purpose was to assess the extent of professional updating, student involvement efforts, use of media, employee education efforts, and classroom-teacher interactions.

Learning in both the cognitive and affective domains was evident. The most significant finding was the positive impact of periodic continuing contact between the educational institution and seminar participants. Group conferences, rather than telephone contact, had a stronger positive influence on project completion and on several other measures of innovation efforts; both were superior to the traditional no-contact arrangement.

The West Region Seminar (Utah State University 1971) was evaluated both by feedback at seminars and by formal written evaluation. Throughout the evaluation, emphasis was placed upon evaluating the seminar and not the participants.

The written evaluation attempted to determine how participants viewed both the various elements of the seminar and the value of what they learned. Several conclusions were drawn from the evaluation:

1. Participants felt the seminar was valuable.
2. Seminar materials were of the right complexity and were valuable.
3. Most participants felt that it would have been valuable to include teachers and administrators as participants in the seminar.
4. Most would be willing to participate in a similar seminar at another time.
5. Most would assist with a food service workshop held in their region.

The four major objectives of the seminar were evaluated in terms of whether they were met "very well," "adequately," or "inadequately." All four objectives were met "very well," according to assessments of between 63 and 78 percent of the directors attending the seminar.

A major USDA conference in 1972 had a twofold purpose: (1) to provide an interchange among state school food service directors, government officials, and cooperating food industry representatives, and (2) to report on findings of the Rutgers USDA/OEO project on school feeding effectiveness (Rutgers University and U.S. Department of Agriculture, Food and Nutrition Service 1972). Proceedings of the conference included reports on the Rutgers research, which had four specific objectives:

1. To design and implement a more effective system of school feeding, especially in schools now without food service facilities.
2. To investigate suitable and economic means of improving the nutritive value and acceptability of school feeding through processing and fortification of donated commodities, and through the use of the technical and marketing ingenuity of the U.S. food industry.
3. To explore and define ways of using school feeding programs to promote the commercial marketing of nutritionally improved foods.
4. To gather basic data on food acceptability and other management information needed to improve the total USDA feeding program.

State directors of school food service were updated with brief reports on various training projects and studies.

In addition to the 1971 nutrition education seminars, several other major training projects were initiated between 1971 and 1975 by USDA/FNS, from funds authorized by PL 91–248. In the 1976 report, the Service summarized seven completed training projects and five in-progress projects (U.S. Department of Agriculture, Food and Nutrition Service 1976).

Two contracts with the state agency in North Carolina were completed. One project, "Food Procurement Television Course for School Food Service Managers," had as an objective: "To provide training in nutrition for school food service managers and supervisors through identification, development and application of skills necessary for quantity bid and specification buying" (U.S. Department of Agriculture, Food and Nutrition Service 1976).

Fifteen thirty-minute, two-inch broadcast tapes in food procurement for school food service managers and supervisors were developed. The programs contained information on budgeting, purchasing, storage, costing, and recordkeeping. The tapes relied heavily on material applicable only to situations in North Carolina, thus limiting nationwide distribution.

The second North Carolina contract had three objectives:

1. To develop standards and/or requirements for certification for food service workers in school in North Carolina.
2. To develop contents for educational courses designed to meet criteria developed.
3. To conduct seminars for training of personnel involved in school food service work and personnel responsible for special food service programs for children.

This last objective was met in the summers of 1973 and 1974, with in-depth analyses of the nutrition needs of North Carolina children; additional training was given during the school year. Participants tested and revised student training manuals which, along with certification standards, were distributed to other states.

Development of the "Food for Youth" television course for teaching nutrition to school food service employees was the overall objective of a large USDA/FNS contract to the New England States Educational Council, Inc. in 1971 (U.S. Department of Agriculture, Food and Nutrition Service 1976). Specifically, the course was developed to: motivate school food service personnel to use existing knowledge and tools to upgrade children's diets; improve their understanding and increase their knowledge of nutrition; and illustrate the significance of nutrition to the growth, development, health, and productivity of the individual.

The content of the course was based on the nutrition education concepts formulated by the Interagency Council on Nutrition Education. Under the terms of the contract, the New England States Educational Council, Inc., in conjunction with WGBH Educational Foundation of Boston and with Harvard School of Public Health, produced the following: ten thirty-minute, high band color videotapes and two dubs of each; a study guide containing discussion questions and quizzes; and a promotion brochure containing information about the series and space for a registration blank to be mailed to the appropriate address within each state.

All facets of the contract were completed satisfactorily, and the finished product was accepted by USDA/FNS in January of 1973.

The series was piloted on television stations in five New England states in January and February of 1973; other states received the series on 16mm film in September 1975. Guidelines for administering the "Food for Youth" series were distributed to the states in January 1976.

Two other major contracts for materials development were awarded in 1973 and 1975 (U.S. Department of Agriculture, Food and Nutrition Service 1976). The University of Wisconsin Extension Service contracted to develop a comprehensive correspondence series for school food service managers, which included eight courses on the following topics: (1) Basic Nutrition and Menu Planning, (2) Food Systems Management and Operation, (3) Quantity Food Purchasing, (4) Quantity Food Preparation, (5) Facility Layout, Equipment Purchase and Use, (6) Nutrition Education, (7) New Trends in Food Service Management and Nutrition, and (8) Interpretations and Implementation of USDA Child Nutrition Legislation and Regulations. Course packets consisted of a series of audio cassette tapes; a study guide containing course objectives, practical on-the-job learning experiences stated in behavioral terms, bibliography of print and audiovisual references, pre- and post-tests, suggested schedule and instructions for use; and supplemental booklets and reading materials.

The other major materials development project was contracted to the American Hotel and Motel Association (U.S. Department of Agriculture, Food and Nutrition Service 1977). The series included eleven manuals on the following topics: (1) Instructor's Guide, (2) Financial Management for Child Nutrition Programs in School, (3) History, Legislation, and Operation of Child Nutrition Programs, (4) Principles and Practices of Resource Management for Child Nutrition Programs, (5) Nutrition and Menu Planning for Child Nutrition Programs, (6) Principles of Equipment and Layout Design for Child Nutrition Programs, (7) Principles of Quantity Food Purchasing, Receiving, and Storage for Child Nutrition Programs, (8) Quantity Food Preparation for Child Nutrition Programs, (9) Merchandising and Public Relations for Child Nutrition Programs, (10) Principles and Practices of Sanitation and Safety in Child Nutrition Programs, and (11) Nutrition Education for Child Nutrition Programs.

The basic format of each training manual provided a series of instructional lessons which could be used to conduct individual training sessions of about one hour. Each lesson focused on a topic of importance within the general subject area. A lesson introduction indicated the overall purpose of the lesson and its objectives; the lesson itself included a content outline, suggested training activities, references for the instructor and participants when additional information is desired, and pre- and post-tests.

In 1973 USDA/FNS cooperated with ASFSA on an Instructor's Institute designed with two objectives: (1) to "teach teachers to teach," and (2) to develop nutrition education training packages (U.S. Department of Agriculture, Food and Nutrition Service 1976). During a one-week session at the University of Oklahoma Center for Continuing Education, participants received instruction in the following areas: (1) Motivation, (2) Establishing Behavioral Objectives, (3) Teaching Techniques, and (4) Effective Use of the Media.

Institute sessions also were devoted to the development of sixteen nutrition education training packages. Participants were encouraged to use the packages in their training programs and to evaluate their usefulness. The following conclusions were drawn from follow-up questionnaires to participants:

1. The institute was of great benefit to most participants.
2. The greatest benefit was the introduction of many new training ideas and techniques.
3. Most participants had incorporated, or planned to incorporate, into their training sessions new ideas gained at the institute.
4. As a result of the institute, many indicated they were more aware of the need for, and planned to become more involved in, nutrition education.

The Five-State Nutrition Education Project has been lauded as a major contribution to the field because of the model provided for team training of school food service personnel and educators (De-Zeeuw 1978). This project represented a cooperative effort of five southern states (Alabama, Florida, Georgia, Mississippi, and Tennessee) to design and test the effectiveness of a team approach to nutrition education. The Georgia Department of Education was the contracting agency.

The project was based on the premise that the classroom is the logical place to learn about nutrition, and the school food service program is the logical laboratory for practice. Because school food service managers and teachers share the responsibility for nutrition education, they were trained as a team to teach nutrition. Their necessary competencies were identified and training modules were developed. The objectives of the project were:

Phase I

1. To identify the competencies needed by teachers and school food service personnel to teach students in grades three to five nutrition education and to provide for inclusion of such competencies in existing catalogs of competencies.
2. To develop training modules on selected competencies to be used to train teachers and school food service personnel.

Phase II

3. To test and evaluate the training modules using pairs of teachers and school food service personnel.
4. To evaluate the effectiveness of using training modules with evaluation tools designed for specific competencies.
5. To publish the list of competencies, the training modules, and the evaluation tools for regional and nationwide use.

The approach to the project was multifaceted:

1. An advisory committee, composed of two persons from each of the participating state agencies, served as the policymaking body of the project.
2. A state consultant committee, composed of persons representing a variety of nutrition-related fields, served as an influential support in making the project successful within their respective states.
3. Other consultants, from universities within the five states, assisted in clarifying concepts of competency-based education and evaluating responses of potential subcontractors to requests for proposals.
4. A subcontractor, selected by the advisory committee, identified the competencies and developed the training modules and evaluation instruments.
5. Auburn University, University of Florida, University of Southern Mississippi, University of Georgia, and Memphis State University offered the field test training for college credit.
6. School food service/manager teams, selected by the advisory committee, participated in the project's field testing.
7. The project director assisted in the development and

evaluation of materials and conducted the field test training and follow-up.

The nutrition content competencies needed by the manager/teacher teams were identified through a national survey of nutrition education experts and the use of three rounds of survey instruments administered to the advisory committee. The committee, in collaboration with the subcontractor, also identified competencies in the areas of interpersonal and instructional skills.

Training modules developed for use in the training sessions were based upon the competencies identified by the advisory committee for implementing the team approach to nutrition education. The modules, which were tested in a one-week training session in each of the five states, emphasized experimental learning in the process of developing a team approach.

Evaluation instruments were administered to the participants during the training session. The effectiveness of the training modules was also evaluated according to the teams' development of action plans for implementation during the school year. A final evaluation came from three follow-up sessions held in each of the five states during the 1974–75 school year. At each session, the project director met with the teams for additional training, retraining, and project evaluation; the director also visited each team in its school to evaluate progress and provide assistance.

The following outcomes resulted from the Five State Nutrition Education Project:

1. Competencies in the areas of nutrition content, interpersonal skills, and instructional skills were identified for manager-teacher teams teaching nutrition education to students in grades three to five.
2. Training modules were developed around the identified competencies for use in training managers and teachers as teams.
3. The training modules were tested and evaluated in each of five states.
4. The evaluation demonstrated the effectiveness of using training modules. Managers and teachers increased both their nutrition content knowledge and their confidence in achieving instructional and interpersonal competencies.
5. The lists of competencies, training modules, and evaluation

tools were disseminated to each of the five participating state education agencies and the regional and Washington offices of the U.S. Department of Agriculture. Each of the five states also designed plans for in-state dissemination of the project's materials and process.

In 1975 five federal grants were awarded to state agencies to assist in identifying competencies of school food service personnel. Grant projects were funded in Maine, New Hampshire, New Jersey, South Dakota, and Wyoming (National Advisory Committee on Child Nutrition 1976).

The New Hampshire project provided funds for a modular certification training program to present to school food service employees and managers in their home regions. The goals of the training were to enable more nutritious meals to be served through the Child Nutrition Programs, to prepare school food service employees to assume a role in educating students about food and nutrition, to increase effectiveness and efficient performance of duties, and to prepare the staff members for greater responsibilities (National Advisory Committee on Child Nutrition, 1979).

The project centered around the development of nine instructional modules designed to provide school food service employees and managers with basic professional skills related to their areas of expertise. The agenda included organizing and training the instructional staff and collecting resources for the project, publicizing the program, recruiting the pilot training class, and conducting and later evaluating the pilot test. A self-contained mobile unit made the training available in all areas of the state (Alonzo 1979).

The New Jersey grant provided funds to identify those areas of competency necessary for school food service personnel to produce meals in compliance with the Child Nutrition Program standards, to develop curriculum packages for these areas, and to evaluate the effectiveness of pilot instruction programs in increasing food service performance. Curricula were developed according to worker responsibility—cook, baker, cashier, lunchroom aide—and used existing school facilities across the state as training sites (National Advisory Committee on Child Nutrition 1979).

The USDA provides important training resources for the Child Nutrition Programs, including such basic operational materials as food-buying, menu-planning, food-storage, and equipment guides, and the quantity recipe set (U.S. Department of Agriculture, Food and Nutrition Service, 1975). The menu-planning and food-buying guides were revised in light of the new lunch pattern in the 1979 regulations (U.S. Department of Agriculture, Food and Nutrition Service 1979).

Another significant resource is the Food and Nutrition Information and Educational Materials Center of the USDA National Agricultural Library (FNIC Literature Search 1979), which was designed to disseminate information for nutrition education and food service training (U.S. Department of Agriculture, Food and Nutrition Service 1973). FNIC is a depository and distribution center for all types of audiovisual and print materials for training and education programs. An evaluation of FNIC was reported in process in the 1978 report of USDA/FNS projects.

State-Level Training

Although the previous section included several federally funded state-level projects, published reports of state-level training programs are limited. In fact, as mentioned earlier, there is a real need for a comprehensive description of state-level training, including surveys and analyses of materials. In the time span surveyed, we found three papers on state-level training, as well as other works previously listed (Luck 1979, Georgia Department of Education 1975, Alonzo 1979). We include here a state-level curriculum developed for junior college programs in California, because it is a widely distributed resource with nationwide applicability (Greig 1978).

Martin (1965), in the mid-1960s, described the Training in Depth program of the Georgia Department of Education. The program was designed to be comprehensive and sequential and to provide the essentials in philosophy, content, skills, and understanding. Martin indicated that the increased training potential was made possible through funds from the Vocational Act of 1963 and the Manpower Development Act.

No training papers were found for the period from the late 1960s to the early 1970s. In 1976 Jenkins and Watts (1976) described training programs in Texas and in South Dakota. Summer workshops were an important part of the training efforts in both of these states. The Texas workshops were limited to cafeteria managers and supervisors and were offered in eight areas of the state. Six three-day courses were taught regularly: basic and advanced management, money management, nutrition, menu planning, and food purchasing. In South Dakota the "Food for Youth" television series developed in New England for personnel training was shown on the state's public television network in 1975 and 1976.

Carlson (1978) described the evolution of a district training program which she initiated as a state-level program in Nebraska. Beginning with development of a set of competencies, the program was divided into units so that individuals received training according to the knowledge and skills needed for their job responsibilities. Eleven courses were offered through a community college in Lincoln, with two class sections meeting weekly throughout the school year. Upon completion of 151 classroom and laboratory hours, employees were awarded state certification.

Greig (1978) briefly described some of the training programs in Kansas, which have been cooperatively planned and provided by the state agency, the local districts, and the land grant universities. Vocational level courses for food service personnel are offered in at least twenty statewide locations, during the year as night courses and during the summer as day courses. These courses are designed to train personnel in food purchasing and preparation, systems management, personnel management, and more recently, basic nutrition. The state office also works in conjunction with the Department of Dietetics, Restaurant and Institutional Management of Kansas State University in offering college credit courses designed for school food service administrators, managers, and teachers.

A report of the early NET Program summarized a few beginning efforts in employee training under the aegis of that program. Tennessee is using the Five-State model to train food service manager-teacher teams; Michigan is showing the "Food for Youth" television series developed in New England for food service personnel training.

The food service education guide developed in California presents another model which has nationwide applicability. Designed through the cooperation of dietitians and school food service professionals, the curriculum guide is a multilevel educational program for training health care or school food service personnel. For both professions, there is a shared curriculum, with only a few specialty courses geared uniquely for school or health care personnel (California Community Colleges 1975).

District-Level Training Efforts

Only a few descriptive reports of district-level training were found in the literature. Program design efforts would be enhanced by a complete catalog of district programs.

Hoglund (1966, 1967) described curriculum development and evaluation for an on-the-job training program for student noon-hour assistants. Operational procedures of various work stations, performance factors, and requisite knowledge were key aspects considered in curriculum design. Self-rating was the primary technique used to evaluate the program.

Dunlap (1971) described a program in Newport News, Virginia, schools in which mentally handicapped students were given job training. The Virginia Department of Vocational Rehabilitation provided funds for the project.

The *School Food Service Journal* published a 1978 special feature on personnel training, including six reports on different approaches in district-level training programs. Applebaum (1978) reported that the program in the Corpus Christi, Texas, schools emphasizes training managers for schools with self-contained kitchens and with satellite operations. Employee training, then, is the responsibility of the manager, although an orientation program is available.

In the schools of Hampton, Virginia, periodic one-day workshops are conducted, using a variety of instructional strategies, such as films, discussion, quizzes, and demonstrations (Lowe 1978).

The Olathe, Kansas, school district held a course for central kitchen employees on fruit and vegetable preparation. Funded partially by state vocational education moneys, the course ran for six weeks, and classes met for three hours, twice each week (Bilotta 1978).

The class was divided into six groups, with participants bringing cookbooks from home for menu ideas. Each group selected three recipes for fruits and vegetables they believed students would eat, enlarged the recipes to serve one hundred, analyzed the cost of each total recipe and each serving, and prepared a food order for the ingredients.

The second class started with laboratory procedures, equipment demonstrations, and technique presentations. Once on their own, participants freely moved from one group to another, questioning and observing; the instructor acted as a facilitator of learning and a resource person. Free time during laboratory periods was spent on a two-week menu plan with calculations of each day's menus. During the last class, students critiqued the quality of instruction, class content, and goal realization, and offered suggestions for future classes. The majority wished to continue with another class as soon as possible.

Working cooperatively with the Title III coordinator in the Wilson County, Tennessee, schools, Hamlett (1978) developed a series of videotapes for employee training. Tape contents included equipment use and care, work simplification, quantity food production procedures (such as shaping yeast breads), and nutrition education techniques.

Two school food service directors reported working with colleges and universities to develop educational programs. Lambreth (1978) negotiated an arrangement with a nearby junior college to design a five-course series on school food service management. Courses were offered in the night program during the school year because of student preferences.

Neill (1978) developed a certificate program in school food service management at California's San Jose University in conjunction with other area district directors. Specific objectives included developing particular management competencies. For example, financial management of school food service systems included both public school finance and computer language. Within the program, organizational and executive management were viewed from the perspective of school food service as part of the total education system. Personnel management training stressed state and local practices, as well as methods of development and evaluation. Production management included quantity production in relation to various delivery systems and purchasing standards for equipment.

According to Neill, the twenty-unit certificate program was the first in California. Ten units of the program were required core courses, such as school food service administration and finance, personnel management, and nutrition standards; the student selected the remaining ten units with guidance from the program director.

Roepke (1978) described a concentrated effort to redefine the school food service program in her district as a nutrition education program, rather than merely a service program. Her objectives were twofold: organize and encourage continuing education of personnel, and renovate the food-serving system. These efforts were stimulated by her participation in the USDA Southwest Region Seminar at Kansas State University in 1971. Her second objective, redesigning the school food service program, was her seminar project for the following school year. She believed that the follow-up sessions were the key to formulating a firm goal and keeping the project on target.*

Employee education was an important aspect of program redefinition. Weekly managers' meetings became concentrated training sessions in management fundamentals, organizational techniques, and basic nutrition information with practical applications. Film loops and training materials were obtained from all available sources. The group took field trips; studied food service systems, both commercial and school; and discussed practical and creative applications for the organization.

The district helped make the training attractive by paying fees and expenses for activities. The entire food service staff was urged to become involved in training programs sponsored by the state department of education, vocational courses for school food personnel, and seminars and meetings designed within the state especially for food service staff. Each fall the district has held in-service training sessions before the school term starts.

Professionalism among members of the American School Food Service Association (ASFSA) has been stressed for all employees, and when ASFSA certification became available for Kansas in 1975, all staff members were urged to become certified and to launch continuing education programs for recertification. Managers and staff were encouraged to take advantage of the college credit short courses designed and offered for school food service personnel during the summer at Kansas State University. The

---

*Roepke was a member of the contact group in the follow-up evaluation of the seminar (Kansas State University 1971; Vaden 1973).

district also paid for the higher level education.

Roepke concluded that the continuing education program was an important aspect of reorienting the school food service program in her district. Changes involved adding a soup-salad-sandwich bar in secondary schools, providing choices in the regular lunch menu, serving special occasion menus, and establishing a student advisory council. Successful implementation was in large part the accomplishment of district school food service personnel.

Programs of the ASFSA

As stated in the 1979 bylaws, one purpose of the American School Food Service Association is to "encourage and develop the highest standards for school food service personnel, by providing appropriate educational programs" (American School Food Service Association 1979). In this section we examine ASFSA's program emphases on personnel training and development during the 1970s.

In 1973 a certification program authorized by the ASFSA executive board was designed as "a means of granting recognition ... for efforts to seek improvement of self and of the profession" (American School Food Service Association 1974). The program was pilot tested in Colorado, Michigan, and North Carolina in 1973–74 and in eleven more states in 1974–75.

Members of the association could be certified in one of three classifications: director/specialist, manager, or assistant. Within each classification, in-grade steps were defined for experience and education ("Follow the Yellow Brick Road ... to Professionalism" 1974). Initially, a three-year certification was granted to those who had been ASFSA members at least one year prior to application. Continuing education hours were required for recertification, with requirements varying from fifteen to forty-five hours during each three-year period, dependent on certification classification (American School Food Service Association 1974).

Since 1975, most state associations have joined the certification program ("Personnel Training: Someone's in the Kitchen" 1978). In 1979 the School Food Service Foundation assumed responsibility for the program, and the criteria were changed to permit non-members to become certified ("Changes Seen in TSFSF Certification Program" 1979). Also, continuing education prerequisites were established; minimum required credits varied with the level of certification ("Certification Program Moves to the Foundation" 1979).

Among the continuing education and professional growth activities of ASFSA in the 1970s was a program designed to encourage association members to take the GED test to gain high school equivalency. Initiated by ASFSA's Ad Hoc Continuing Education Committee in 1972, the program was developed in response to the finding that 40 percent of the employees in school food service did not have a high school education or equivalent (American School Food Service Association 1973, "G[reat] E[ducation] D[eal]," 1974). A second major task of the committee was development of course recommendations for school food service training programs in two-year colleges (American School Food Service Association 1973).

"Train the Trainer" was the focus of two institutes sponsored by ASFSA in cooperation with the University of Oklahoma in 1973 and Kansas State University in 1976 (Caton 1976). The 1973 institute emphasized adult education concepts. USDA also cooperated with ASFSA by providing a grant to fund the expenses of twenty-five school food service directors attending the institute (National Advisory Council on Child Nutrition 1974). Objectives and outcomes were discussed in the previous section of this paper on USDA training efforts.

The second institute in 1976 emphasized planning, coordination, and conduct of instructional programs for school food service personnel (Caton 1976). Competency-based education, a topic selected as an outgrowth of the work of the ASFSA Certification Committee, was the key focus of the discussions and group work sessions. Attended by approximately fifty persons, presentations focused on principles of adult education, competency-based education, interpersonal communication, teaching resources, and creativity in teaching. Participants developed competency-based lesson plans appropriate to the training needs in their own district school food service programs.

Beginning in 1975, the ASFSA Certification Committee placed major emphasis on identifying competencies needed by school food service personnel to strengthen the certification program. Six major areas of expertise were identified for competency definition: customer services, nutrition, financial control, quality control, productivity planning, and supervision (Caton 1976). Those efforts culminated in the 1978 publication of recommended competencies for school nutrition program personnel (American School Food Service Association 1978). The committee defined job functions and competencies for the certification program's three classifications of district-level personnel and suggested that the competencies be used to develop and revise educational programs for school food service personnel.

Among components of a professional growth system delineated to implement the competencies were the following:

1. Job descriptions—including minimum educational/experience requirements, classification levels, salary ranges, and performance expectations.
2. Staffing pattern recommendations.
3. Education system—involving formal and informal educational opportunities, cooperatively planned and administered by professional associations, educational institutions, and state agencies.
4. System of evaluation—including assessment of training needs as well as development of instruments and techniques to measure competency attainment.
5. Reward system—including recognition, career advancement opportunities, and salary increments.

The commitment of ASFSA to professional growth programs was reaffirmed at the 1976 Decade Planning Seminar in Vail, Colorado. Two of the goals endorsed to guide the association's work were directly related to human resources development in school food service: (1) to expand and develop ASFSA's professional growth framework, and (2) to establish educational requirements and competencies for school food service positions at all levels.

Each year the AFSFA president-elect is responsible for reviewing the existing program of work and the long-range plan of the association for the purpose of developing a program for his or her term as president (American School Food Service Association 1979). All the reviews of the last decade emphasize continuing education and professional growth of the membership. In the 1980–81 program of work President-elect Nix again emphasized the goals of strengthening certification and encouraging professional growth (Nix 1980).

University Research Related to School Food Service Personnel Training

Reports from university research were categorized as surveys of programs; materials development; or development, testing, and evaluation of specific training approaches, methodologies, or programs. Most of the reports selected for review were concerned with training for school food service personnel; however, a few relevant studies in other segments of institutional food service were also selected.

Surveys.   Two studies reviewed were surveys of the types of training used in selected areas. Young (1966) queried a random sample of school food service directors in Massachusetts and New York about nonsupervisory employee training. With 43 percent of the sample responding, results indicated that the methods and procedures were of limited use, and orientations for new personnel were held infrequently. Informal on-the-job training was the most common method reported, few training aids were used, and evaluations were limited.

Hunyadi (1972) investigated the types of training used in Ohio school food service systems, using a mail questionnaire sent to school food service directors. She also studied the relationship between training procedures and labor costs. Almost half of the respondents reported there were no training programs in their systems. Nutrition education, student participation, and federal program requirements were considered the weakest aspects of programs. By correlating evaluation scores, she found that labor costs and training were unrelated; data for the analysis, however, were limited.

Materials Development.   Apparently a strong need existed to define program policies and procedures in the late 1950s and early 1960s. Four master's theses completed during that period had as their objective the development of policy manuals for food service personnel. Brown (1957) and Wathan (1960) developed employee manuals for local district programs; Baumberger (1962) and Clark (1962) collaborated to design a state manual for managers and cook managers in Ohio. While all four of these developmental research projects surveyed literature and various experts in the field, none of the papers reported evaluation of the completed manual.

Cui (1968) designed a teaching guide on motivation for a five-session, in-service training seminar for food service supervisors. The guide included objectives, content outlines, and visual material for each lesson. Again, the project did not include evaluation of the guide's effectiveness.

In another developmental project, Oyer (1960) developed a nutrition education test to assess school food service workers' knowledge and understanding of nutrition as well as the relationship between menu planning for quantity food production and nutrient content of food. With a split-half reliability coefficient of .65, the test appeared to have some ability to discriminate: a positive relationship was found between test performance and education level. The author recommended further refinement before use as both a diagnostic and training evaluation tool.

Specific Training Approaches, Methodologies, and Programs. In the design at one project, Mullan (1965) investigated coordinating high school-level vocational education for supervised food service workers with the school lunch program. Three alternative plans were developed and evaluated by an expert panel:

Plan I: One-semester program for senior high students during which no other courses were scheduled.

Plan II: Two class periods per day for two semesters for juniors or seniors. The first semester was a food preparation laboratory, and the second, supervised work experience.

Plan III: Two-year program for junior and senior years, with two semesters of food preparation and two of supervised work experience.

The panel consensus was that Plans II and III were superior to Plan I.

Several studies concerned the evaluation of short-term educational experiences, such as summer workshops. Since concentrated training strategies are a common method of training in school service, we considered these studies particularly relevant.

In 1955 Ewing evaluated a series of two-day school lunch workshops sponsored by the state agency in West Virginia. Eight workshops, held at locations throughout the state, covered five subject areas selected through a survey of local school personnel: nutrition, food purchasing and menu planning, food preparation, school lunch as part of the total school program, and care and use of equipment.

Approximately three months after the workshops, participants were mailed evaluation surveys. A selected sample of food service personnel who did not attend also were surveyed to determine reasons for nonattendance. Reports indicated favorable reactions and some degree of carryover into job performance from participation in workshops; for example, 70 percent of the cooks had used one or more recipes received at the workshop. One component, the broad-based planning approach involving input from a wide group of potential attendees, appeared to contribute to the success of the workshops.

To evaluate a one-week school lunch training institute sponsored by the New York state agency, Ford (1958) developed two questionnaires: one to be completed by cook and cook/manager workshop participants, and the second by the administrators at the schools where participants were employed. The participant questionnaire evaluated the training institute; the administrator survey secured information about operational improvements observed as a result of the cook's or cook/manager's workshop attendance. Suggestions for future training, particularly food preparation and service, were noted by the administrators.

Between 1967 and 1969, researchers at Iowa State University conducted a comprehensive evaluation of an experimental training program for school food service personnel. The overall objective was to determine the impact of in-service training and certain factors related to effectiveness. The following topics were included in the three one-week courses: food preparation, supervision, menu making, type-A lunch, record keeping, nutrition, purchasing, sanitation, school-community relations, work methods, and philosophy of school lunch.

Knauf (1967); Bunge, McKinley, and Montag (1969); and Ninemeier, McKinley, and Montag (1970) constructed subject matter evaluation instruments to measure cognitive learning resulting from the training. Results reported by Bunge, McKinley, and Montag substantiated the potential worth of short-term training for learning facts and applying generalizations.

Ninemeier, McKinley, and Montag analyzed aptitude learning from on-the-job and other experiences and short-term retention.

Three groups of school lunch employees participated in the study: a one-year experimental group, a three-year experimental group, and a control group. The one-year and control groups each consisted of forty-three persons, while thirty-five participants comprised the three-year group. The one-year experimental group attended all three short courses in one summer; the three-year group had attended two short courses in previous years and attended the third during the experiment; the control group did not attend any of the short courses. The criteria used in selecting the groups were length of experience in food service (seven years and under or eight years and over); level of formal education (grade eleven or less and grade twelve or more); and job responsibility (cook and manager). Using the General Aptitude Test Battery (GATB) as the aptitude measure, the researchers found no relationship between GATB scores and gain in job knowledge due to training, implying that the training was likely to be as beneficial to persons with low aptitudes as to those with high aptitudes.

Simons measured the job performance of a sample of trainees to determine if a relationship existed between what was learned in training and practices on the job. Specific objectives were to:

1. Compare the on-the-job performance of trained and control groups.
2. Relate on-the-job performance to posttest scores.
3. Determine the extent to which the trained group translated job knowledge, as reflected by specific test items, into action.
4. Relate on-the-job performance to aptitudes.
5. Compare retention of learning between trained and control groups in the subject matter area of nutrition.

The sample consisted of twenty-four school lunch managers from the one-year experimental and control groups, selected on the basis of posttest scores. An instrument of performance measures was constructed to rate on-the-job behavior. The basic training program learnings reflected in the evaluation instruments became the basis for the performance measures. Each measure was preclassified according to one of the eleven subject matter areas covered in the short course. Designed to obtain data by such techniques as direct observation, directive interview, and inspection, the measures were administered on a trial basis in three schools. After the performance measures were developed, they were administered in all twenty-four schools by two observers who spent a full work day in each school. Following the performance measures, participants were retested on selected items from the subject–matter evaluation instruments for nutrition and philosophy of school lunch.

The findings were significant for only one subject-matter area, Type-A lunch. Why other subject-matter areas were not significant could be ascribed to the training program itself, lack of retention or insufficient motivation on the part of the trainees, the design of the experiment, and variables that were difficult to control.

Benedict (1969) analyzed subjective ratings of the participants' performance on the job and perceptions of training. Ratings from the school administrators and from participants were obtained by means of a written questionnaire; information from two subordinates of each of twelve managers in the experimental group was obtained by interview. Eight months after training, the administrators, subordinates, and trainees were asked to cite specific examples of change in the operation of the school lunch program which were (and were not) attributable to the trainees' participation in the short courses. Behavorial changes most frequently cited as attributable to the short courses were:

Observes various techniques that result in more appealing menus.

Uses improved work methods.

Supervises workers better.

Applies various principles of food preparation learned in the short courses.

Exhibits improved attitudes.

Effects changes in menu to better meet requirements of Type-A lunch.

Makes better use of government commodities.

Shows deeper concern about controlling food costs.

Shows more willingness to exert leadership.

Implements better sanitation practices.

Keeps better records.

Eight months after training, administrators of both the managers and cooks, as well as the cooks themselves, reported a positive attitude change. Based on this finding, coupled with the fact that a large number of participants referred to philosophy of school lunch as one of the most helpful aspects of training, it was concluded that trainees gained a better understanding of their relationship to the school lunch program and became more self-reliant and responsible. The relatively high percentage of managers who made changes in job performance, together with parallel ratings of change by administrators, subordinates, and the trainees themselves, is further evidence that the training program produced change.

The findings in this report suggest that learning during short courses cannot be adequately assessed by pretests or on-the-job performance measurements alone. Ratings were found to be more discerning than objective evaluative devices for the measurement of intangible outcomes of training. It was concluded that subjective measurements are a particularly useful tool when used in conjunction with pre- and post-tests and objective measurements of on-the-job performance.

In another assessment of short-term training, Curry and Toma (1975) examined the relationship between level of nutrition education knowledge and participation in certification classes. Based on responses to a seventy-point true/false questionnaire, they reported that participants scored higher than nonparticipants.

Spears described evaluations of two summer short courses for school food service personnel. The first (1973) was a team learning approach for personnel with different educational and experience backgrounds. The crux of the method was the utilization of a single functional concept for the course topic and division of the class into small learning teams, each representing the diversity of the class. The topic for the course was purchasing, a function which all the students had some experience with in their jobs. An intensive one-week course was planned, with enrollment open to all school food service personnel. The award of graduate credit for those qualified was predicated on a daily seminar conducted by the instructor. Twelve students were registered for graduate credit, twelve for undergraduate credit, and one was a special student. All reading materials, as well as self-study units, were available in the department media center. Approximately half the class were managers and half directors. Teams of managers and directors worked on a purchasing project. The graduate seminar was on materials management applications to school food service operations.

In end-of-course evaluations, most of the participants indicated a preference for one topic in depth rather than briefer treatment of several topics. Most preferred one-week rather than two-week sessions, with possible topics for future courses in personnel management, nutrition education, employee training, and quantity food production. Spears concluded that the team approach was a method well suited to the needs of school food service personnel.

Spears's second paper (1978) was a report of a one-week "train the trainer" short course designed to prepare teachers for the thirty-six-hour summer vocational classes for school food service employees sponsored by the Kansas Department of Education (KSU). Content and format of the course were patterned after the ASFSA-KSU–sponsored institute described above, in which competency-based education was a central theme (Caton 1976). Cognitive and affective evaluations were used. The knowledge score showed a mean increase of 27 percent. The semantic differential approach used for affective assessment indicated no change from pre- to post-test.

Three reports of evaluations of work simplification training were found. Armstrong (1960) described the development of a work simplification training program. Swigert (1965) developed a series of transparencies for employee training in the principles of motion economy and presented them to twelve school food service personnel. A questionnaire completed by participants, an informal conference, and observations to assess work habit changes were the evaluation strategies.

Beard (1970) used work sampling to evaluate school food service employees' performance before and after a training program on work simplification principles. Although the results were not definitive, Beard concluded that his approach had potential as a training evaluation technique.

Blacksten (1968) developed a programmed instruction unit for training employees in the operation of the dish machine; he used a linear type instruction in the booklet. The lesson was administered four different times to groups of three trainees, who suggested revisions for the booklet. The author suggested further investigations into the effectiveness of programmed instruction for food service employees.

Sumbingco (1976) developed a programmed textbook to teach two tasks, a relatively simple one (portioning and serving pie) and a difficult one (cleaning a food slicer). Evaluation with eleven food service employees indicated that the materials were effective for learning and retention, and that the employees had positive reactions to the approach.

Several studies compared the value of two techniques for training. For example, a series of four projects completed at Kansas State University and two at Iowa State University focused on the comparative efficacy of various training strategies.

Kahl (1968) compared two methods for presenting a visual instruction program to food service employees; he developed a slide series on preparing a flight-type dish machine for operation. In Method I instruction was given in the dish room; in Method II subjects were instructed in another room without the machine. Evaluation included comparison of instruction time, trial time, and number of errors. Both methods were effective, although Method I was somewhat superior. Method I required more of the instructor's time and a special setup.

Holle (1969) determined the effectiveness of an individual slide study method versus a group lecture method for teaching sanitation. She concluded that the program was effective when presented by either method; the one advantage of the slide method was the fact that it was self-instructional.

Frame (1971) developed training programs for two food preparation procedures—breading/deep frying and making sliced meat sandwiches—to use with a videotape recorder and a training manual. The criterion for determining the effectiveness of the training media was the number of steps performed correctly two weeks after the training. Videotape instruction was found to be somewhat superior to the training manual for teaching the defined tasks.

Scharf (1972) compared two forms of instruction for presenting an orientation program on sanitation to new food service workers, a programmed text and a lecture-transparency presentation. Both methods were effective in teaching cognitive concepts, but the programmed text offered the advantage of not requiring an instructor's time.

Acacio, McKinley, and Scruggs (1972) compared the merits of programmed instruction and group training. The specific objectives of this study were to (1) develop a self-instructional program for food service personnel for three subject matter areas—nutrition, Type-A lunch, and menumaking—using programmed instruction; (2) determine whether there were differences in pre- and post-training job knowledge among the groups studied; (3) relate pre- and post-training job knowledge to the trainees' length of experience in food service and educational level; and (4) evaluate the self-instructional package objectively and subjectively.

Three groups of school food service managers participated in the study: (1) a self-instruction group, which received programmed instruction administered as a home study course, (2) a short course group, trained by attending three five-day short courses on the Iowa State University campus; and (3) a control group, which received no training during the experiment.

The researchers concluded that the training provided by programmed instruction or by the short courses resulted in a gain in job knowledge. The self-instructional package and the short course training were equally effective methods of training food service employees in the selected subject matter areas, as measured by the subject matter evaluation instruments. The advantages identified for group training were sharing of experiences among learners; interaction between instructor and learner; and more effective communication through seeing, hearing, and discussion. The effectiveness of group training may be limited, however, by the lack of qualified instructors in the area of food service. In addition, scheduling of group training programs that will not disrupt ongoing food service activities may be difficult. Group training that requires the learners to travel to training centers may create problems for individuals having to be away from home.

A key advantage identified for programmed instruction was the opportunity for self-pacing, enabling the individual to progress through the instructional material at his or her own rate of learning and performance. Training sessions can be arranged to meet individual scheduling needs, and programmed instruction can be used alone or integrated with other training programs. Management can reach employees who are widely dispersed at home or at work without arranging for group presentations. The participants disliked some aspects of the self-instructional program: interruptions while studying at home, absence of an instructor to explain material that was not understood, and the need to learn how to study.

In another comparative study, Rinke, Brown, and McKinley (1975) investigated the effectiveness of two methods of presenting a short training program on selected aspects of food service sanitation. One method, live instruction, consisted of 35 mm slides presented with comments and questions by an instructor and an opportunity for participants to respond. The second method was taped instruction, in which the same slides, comments, and questions were presented as a synchronized slide-tape program, without an instructor.

The major objectives of the program were to instruct participants in the characteristics of bacteria, methods to control bacteria, and concepts of sanitation. The training program was evaluated and revised on several occasions, with the final program presented in two parts on different days. As measured by a paper-and-pencil evaluation, both the live and taped methods of instruction were effective for training food production employees in sanitation.

CONCLUSION AND RECOMMENDATIONS

We reviewed literature published during the last twenty-five years on significant developments influencing the training of school food service personnel, on training needs in school food service, and on development and/or evaluation of training materials and programs. We also examined selected literature on training in other aspects of the institutional food service field, if deemed to have direct applicability to school food service. Published reports of federal, state, and district training efforts, programs of the American School Food Service Association, and studies related to development and/or evaluation of training materials and programs evolving from university research efforts were included in this chapter.

How far has the field come in meeting the recommendations or rectifying the problems identified in these various reports issued since the early days of the program? Diversity of participants, scarcity of qualified instructors, broad scope of subject matter, and limited evaluation and follow-up were identified as problems hindering the training programs of the 1940s and 1950s. Although progress appears to have been made, these problems still exist to some extent, especially inadequate evaluation of training efforts.

The need for personnel standards, including educational and experience requirements, has been underscored in position statements and reports issued since the 1940s by various study and advisory groups. To date, program regulations do not address personnel standards for the child nutrition programs, although many other federal programs, such as Medicare and WIC, specify personnel qualifications for direction and supervision of programs.

The 1967 School Lunch Task Force recommended that regional seminars be held periodically for state and district staff, that graduate traineeships be developed, that programs be expanded in vocational schools and junior colleges for unit manager and personnel training, and that a national materials center be established. The USDA regional seminar program initiated in 1969 was discontinued in 1971, even though available reports indicated that evaluations were generally positive. There has been some progress in vocational and junior/community college program development, according to reports on state and district efforts. Establishment of the FNIC in response to recommendations by the task force and other groups (for example, the National Advisory Council on Child Nutrition) is a considerable accomplishment. However, the recommended establishment of graduate traineeships for educating supervisory personnel has received little attention.

The need to upgrade personnel in school food service has been among the major recommendations of the National Advisory Council on Child Nutrition since its inception in 1971. In its first report the council recommended that competencies be developed, personnel standards and qualifications be established, and curricula for pre- and in-service training and a manual for program operations be developed. Training for instructional staff was another early recommendation. Some progress has been made by USDA and other groups; however, these efforts still require emphasis. For example, the national study profiling school food service personnel indicated that only three out of every ten employees had attended a training session in the last ten years, although about half of the survey group desired more training.

From this review, we draw the following conclusions and recommendations concerning school food service personnel training:

1. Personnel standards should be developed for various levels of personnel at the local, district, and state levels, including qualifications for education and experience to insure program direction and operation by competent staff.

2. Work by various groups on development of competencies should be continued, and the competencies developed should be validated through combined efforts of practition-

ers and educators. These competencies should be the basis for developing education and training models for all levels of personnel.

3. A more systematic approach to education and training is needed, using competencies as the beginning point.

4. Evaluation strategies for all types of training at all levels should be strengthened, with emphasis on assessment of learning in all domains and changes in performance. Evaluations have too often focused on reactions to a training program and setting rather than on the learner and the transfer of learning to improved performance.

5. Greater use of the FNIC should be encouraged, especially as a depository and dissemination system for district- and state-level education and training materials.

6. Comprehensive surveys of state and district education and training programs and materials are needed, with emphasis on identification of effective models.

7. Stronger alliances with institutions of higher education are needed. Undergraduate and graduate programs should be developed for the education of state and district supervisory personnel. Curricula should include courses in nutrition, child development, nutrition education, food science, food service management, and school administration. Competencies in these areas are needed for effective administration of a comprehensive school food service and nutrition education program. Practicums in school food service administration should be included at both the undergraduate and graduate levels.

8. The regional seminar program should be reactivated as continuing education for state and district administrative personnel. Seminars should be held every two to three years in each region, preferably at land grant colleges or state universities with expertise and programs in nutrition and food service management. A cooperative program-planning model should be used, with input from federal, regional, state, and district personnel and university faculty. Evaluation strategies should include follow-up contact and reinforcement to encourage implementation of learned concepts appropriate to participants' school food service programs.

9. Revision of the materials developed under the two major

contracts of USDA/FNS (the manuals developed at AHMA and the correspondence course) and an effective dissemination system should be priorities of USDA.

10. Major evaluations of existing certification programs (ASFSA and the state programs) should be undertaken, including assessment of the various continuing education requirements in effecting changes in job performance.

11. USDA should increase efforts to work cooperatively with state agencies, the higher education community, and professional associations, in developing education and training priorities, models, and directions for the child nutrition programs.

BIBLIOGRAPHY

Abt Associates Inc. 1979. Evaluation of the Nutrition Education and Training Program Administered by the U.S. Department of Agriculture, Food and Nutrition Service. RFP no. 12–FNS–79. Volume I: Technical Proposal. Cambridge, Mass.: Abt Associates Inc., April 16.

Acacio, F.B.; McKinley, M.M.; and Scruggs, M. 1972. Self-Instructional Program of Training for Food Service Personnel Compared with Group Training. *J. Home Econ.* 64:39.

Alonzo, R.S. 1979. School Food Service Training Takes to the Road. *School Food Service J.* 33:48, 52.

American School Food Service Association. 1974. *ASFSA Certification Handbook.* Denver: American School Food Service Association.

American School Food Service Association, Continuing Education Committee. 1973. *Course Recommendations for School Food Service Training Programs in Two-Year Colleges.* Denver: American School Food Service Association.

Appelbaum, G. 1978. Persistence + Determination = Success. *School Food Service J.* 32:50.

Armstrong, P.R. 1960. *A Training Program in Work Simplification.* Master's thesis, Kansas State University.

Baumberger, H.R. 1962. *A Proposed Manual for Managers and Cook-Managers of Federal Supported Lunch Programs in Ohio, Part I.* Master's thesis, Ohio State University.

Beard, V.B. 1970. *Work Sampling as a Method of Evaluating a School Food Service Training Program.* Master's thesis, University of Tennessee.

Benedict, J.M. 1969. *Subjective Evaluation of an Experimental Training Program for Food Service Personnel.* Master's thesis, Iowa State University.

Bilotta. 1978. Try It! You'll Like It! *School Food Service J.* 32:54.

Blacksten, P.A. 1968. *Programmed Instruction for Training Food Service Workers in Dishmachine Operation.* Master's thesis, University of Washington.

Boudreaux, L.J. 1972. *A Study Concerning Academic and Experience Requirements for School Food Service Supervisory Personnel.* Master's thesis, University of Southern Mississippi.

Brown, D.A. 1957. *The Development of a Training Program for the*

School Lunchroom Employees in the Pasadena Independent School District. Master's thesis, University of Houston.

Bunge, M.M.; McKinley, M.M.; and Montag, G.M. 1969. An Experimental Training Program for Food Service Personnel. *J. Home Econ.* 61:433.

Bylaws: American School Food Service Association. 1979. Denver: American School Food Service Association.

California Community Colleges, Chancellor's Office. 1975. *A Guide for Foodservice Education* (August).

Carlson, H. 1978. Where Do We Begin? *School Food Service J.* 32:80.

Caton, J. 1976. *Competency-Based Education for School Food Service Personnel, Why and How.* Denver: American School Food Service Association.

Certification Program Moves to the Foundation. 1979. *School Food Service J.* 33:16.

Changes Seen in TSFSF Certification Program. 1979. *School Food Service J.* 33:12.

Childers, J.A. 1961. *The Need of Competent Supervision for Local School Lunch Programs.* Master's thesis, University of Mississippi.

Clark, C.W. 1962. *A Proposed Manual for Managers and Cook-Managers of Federal Supported Lunch Programs in Ohio, Part II.* Master's thesis, Ohio State University.

Clarke, B.L. 1966. *An Investigation of the Knowledge and Managerial Abilities of Mississippi School Lunch Managers.* Master's thesis, University of Southern Mississippi.

Claycombe, W.W.; Bird, J.M.; and Bennett, M.L. 1976. An Evaluation of Supervisory Skills to Determine Training Needs. *Personnel J.* 55:116.

Cui, E.M. 1968. *Teaching Guide on Motivation of Employees for Non-Professional Foodservice Supervisors.* Master's thesis, Kansas State University.

Curry, M., and Toma, R. 1975. Working and Learning in School Foodservice. *School Food Service J.* 26:66.

DeZeeuw, M.L. 1978. Taking the Team Approach to Nutrition Education. *School Food Service J.* 32:48.

Dunlap, D. 1971. All Benefit from Handicaps' Training. *School Food Service J.* 26:83.

Ewing, W.M. 1956. *Evaluation of School Lunch Workshops Spon-*

sored by State Department of Education, School Lunch Division, West Virginia, 1955. Master's thesis, West Virginia University.

Federal Work Agency, Work Projects Administration. 1940. *Operation of School Lunch Projects.* WPA Technical Series, Welfare Circular no. 1. Washington, D.C.: Work Projects Administration.

Fisher, D.E. 1955. *Identification of Supervisory Improvement Needs in the Development of a Training Program for Lunchroom Managers in a School Lunch Program.* Master's thesis, Michigan State University.

Flanagan, T.G. 1971. School Food Services. In *Education in the States: Nationwide Development Since 1900.* Washington, D.C.: National Education Association.

Flanagan, T.G., and Martin, J. 1967. *School Food Service Policies and Standards.* 3rd ed. Tallahassee: Southern States Work Conference on Educational Problems.

Florida Agricultural and Mechanical University, Department of Home Economics. 1971. *Proceedings of the Nutrition Education Seminar: Materials and Methods in Nutrition Education* (July).

FNIC Literature Search. 1979. Nutrition Education. Beltsville, Maryland: Food and Nutrition Information and Education Resources Center, National Agric. Library (November 29).

Follow the Yellow Brick Road . . . to Professionalism. 1974. *School Food Service J.* 28:85.

Ford, A.S. 1958. *An Evaluation of a Training School for School Lunch Personnel in New York State.* Master's thesis, Cornell University.

Frame, C.J. 1971. *A Comparison of Programmed Instructional Methods for Training Foodservice Workers.* Master's thesis, Kansas State University.

Garrett, P.W., and Vaden, A.G. 1978. Influence of Student-Selected Menus on Participation, Plate Waste, and Student Attitudes. *School Food Service Res. Rev.* 2:28.

Garvue, R.J.; Flanagan, T.G.; and Castine, W.H. 1971. *The National School Food Service and Nutrition Education Finance Project.* Special Study no. 8 of the National Educational Finance Project. Supported by the U.S. Department of Agriculture; administered by the Florida Department of Education in cooperation with Florida State University.

Georgia Department of Education. 1975. *The Development and Evaluation of Performance Based Training for Elementary*

Teachers and School Food Service Personnel in Nutrition Educa-tion. Five-State Nutrition Education Project, Final Report (October). Washington, D.C.: U.S. Department of Agriculture, Food and Nutrition Service.

Gibson, J.N., and Scoular, F.I. 1962. Job Stability in Dallas School Lunchrooms. *Am. Dietet. Assoc.* 47:753.

Goertz, G. 1969. School Lunch Task Force Report. In *Proceedings of Southeastern Regional Seminar for School Food Service Administrators.* College of Home Economics, University of Tennessee.

G(reat) E(ducation) D(eal), Have You Finished High School? Would You Like To? 1974. *School Food Service J.* 28:100.

Greig, S. 1978. Nutrition Education in School Foodservice in Kansas. *Am. Dietet. Assoc.* 73:122.

Gunderson, G.W. 1971. *The National School Lunch Program. Background and Development.* FNS 63. Washington, D.C.: U.S. Department of Agriculture, Food and Nutrition Service.

Gunn, M. 1966. *Attitudes of the School Lunch Manager.* Master's thesis, University of Southern Mississippi.

Hamlett, J.E. 1978. Tune into Training. *School Food Service J.* 32:56.

Harwood, V.E., and Brown, H.I. 1968. Labor Turnover in Hospital Dietary Departments. *Am. Dietet. Assoc.* 53:348.

Helber, D.D. 1964. *The Qualifications of School Lunch Directors in the State of Washington.* Master's thesis, University of Washington.

Hoglund, V. 1966. The School Cafeteria—A Training Program. Part I: Curriculum Development for Training Noon-Hour Assistants. *Sch. Lunch J.* 20:70.

———. 1967. The School Lunchroom—A Training Program. Part II: Evaluation for On-the-Job Training in a School Lunchroom. *Sch. Lunch J.* 21:52.

Holle, J.A. 1969. *Development of a Training Program in Sanitation for Foodservice Personnel.* Master's thesis, Kansas State University.

Hopkins, D.E.; Vaden, A.G.; and Vaden, R.E. 1979. Some Determinants of Work Performance in Food Service Systems: Job Satisfaction and the Work Values of School Foodservice Personnel. *J. Am. Dietet. Assoc.* 75:640.

———. 1980. Some Aspects of Organization Identification Among

School Food Service Employees. *School Food Service Res. Rev.* 4:34.

Hospital Continuing Education Project. 1970. *Training and Continuing Education.* Chicago: Hospital Research and Education Trust.

Hunyadi, O.L. 1972. *A Profile of Training Programs for Supervisory Personnel in School Lunch Programs in Ohio.* Master's thesis, Kent State University.

Information Planning Associates, Inc. 1977. *A Profile of School Food Service Personnel.* Contract no. 12–35–600–254. Washington, D.C.: U.S. Department of Agriculture, Food and Nutrition Service (Feb.).

————. 1978. Profile of School Food Service Personnel: Executive Summary. *School Food Service Res. Rev.* 2:34.

Jenkins, D.D., and Watts, M. 1976. Training is Important. *Food and Nutrition* 6 (Oct.): 4.

Joint Committee of the American Dietetic Association, the American School Food Service Association, and the American Home Economics Association. 1949. Recommended Standards for the Selection of Personnel Responsible for the Supervision and Management of the School Lunch Program. *School Food Service News* 6 (Jan.–Feb.):33.

Kahl, K.W. 1968. *Evaluation of Two Visual Presentations of a Training Program for Foodservice Workers.* Master's thesis, Kansas State University.

Kansas State University, College of Home Economics, Department of Institutional Management. 1971. *Proceedings of the Southwest Region School Food Service Seminar: Innovative Approaches to Nutrition Education and Related Management Processes,* ed. A. Vaden (July).

Kende, G.F. et al. 1980. Nutrition Education and Training Needs of Michigan School Food Service Directors and Supervisors. *School Food Service Res. Rev.* 4:27.

Knauf, K. 1967. *Development of an Instrument to Evaluate the Effect of a School Lunch Training Program.* Master's thesis, Iowa State University.

Lambreth,. 1978. Training Tactics. *School Food Service J.* 32:81.

Lester, R.S. 1973. Training Research: Identification of Training Needs. *Personnel J.* 52:180.

Lowe, B. 1978. Move to the Head of the Class. *School Food Service J.* 32:53.

Luck, J. 1979. NET: What's It All About? *School Food Service J.* 33:52.

Martin, J. 1965. Training in Depth: The Georgia School Food Service Training Program. *School Lunch J.* 19:30.

―――. 1978. School Nutrition Programs in Perspective. *J. Am. Dietet. Assoc.* 73:389.

Mullan, L.M. 1965. *Vocational Food Service Education and the School Lunch Program.* Master's thesis, Iowa State University.

National Advisory Council on Child Nutrition. 1972. Annual Report/1971. Washington, D.C.: U.S. Department of Agriculture, Food and Nutrition Service.

―――. 1973. Annual Report/1972. Washington, D.C.: U.S. Department of Agriculture, Food and Nutrition Service.

―――. 1974. Annual Report/1973. Washington, D.C.: U.S. Department of Agriculture, Food and Nutrition Service.

―――. 1975. Fifth Annual Report/1974. Washington, D.C.: U.S. Department of Agriculture, Food and Nutrition Service.

―――. 1976. Annual Report/1975. Washington, D.C.: U.S. Department of Agriculture, Food and Nutrition Service.

―――. 1979. 1977 Annual Report. Washington, D.C.: U.S. Department of Agriculture, Food and Nutrition Service.

Neill. 1978. Management ABCs. *School Food Service J.* 32:52.

Newell, G.E. 1976. How to Plan a Training Program. *Personnel J.* 55:220.

Ninemeier, J.D.; McKinley, M.M.; and Montag, G.M. 1970. Aptitudes in Selection and Training of Food Service Personnel. *J. Am. Dietet. Assoc.* 57:341.

Nix, M. 1980. *The 80s—A Decade for Winning.* Denver: American School Food Service Association.

Nutrition Education and Training Status Reports. 1976. Completed Projects. Washington, D.C.: U.S. Department of Agriculture, Food and Nutrition Service.

Oklahoma State University, College of Home Economics, Department of Food, Nutrition and Institution Administration. 1970. *Proceedings of Southwestern Regional Seminar for School Food Service Administrators* (June).

Oyer, E.J. 1960. The Development of a Nutrition Education Test for School Lunch Personnel. *School Lunch J.* 14:33.

Pelto, J.M., and Sweatt, G.E. 1965. Personnel Turnover in Departments of Dietetics. *J. Am. Dietet. Assoc.* 46:369.

Pennsylvania State University, College of Human Development, Department of Food Service and Housing Administration. 1971. *Proceedings of the Northeast Regional Seminar for School Food Service Supervisors,* ed. S. J. Clemen (July).

Personnel Training: Someone's in the Kitchen. 1978. *School Food Service J.* 32:46.

Proceedings: Planning for the Decade Ahead, A National Seminar. 1976. Denver: American School Food Service Association.

Program Evaluation Status Reports. 1978. Completed Studies. Washington, D.C.: U.S. Department of Agriculture, Food and Nutrition Service.

Public Law 79–396, 79th Congress. 1946. 60 Stat. 231.

Public Law 91–248, 91st Congress. 1970. 84 Stat. 207.

Public Law 94–105, 94th Congress. 1975. 89 Stat. 511.

Public Law 95–166, 95th Congress. 1977. 91 Stat. 1325.

Recommended Competencies for School Nutrition Program Personnel. 1978. Denver: American School Food Service Association.

Riggs, J.M. 1956. *Instruction in Quantity Food Production Integrated with High School Lunch Programs.* Master's thesis, Iowa State College.

Rinke, W.J.; Brown, N.E.; and McKinley, M.M. 1975. Two Methods for Instruction Personnel about Foodservice Sanitation. *J. Am. Dietet. Assoc.* 67:364.

Roepke, R. 1978. Innovations in School Foodservice to Promote Nutrition Education. *J. Am. Dietet. Assoc.* 73:125.

Rutgers University and USDA Food and Nutrition Service. 1972. *Proceedings of the National School Food Service Conference* (June).

Scharf, S.A. 1972. *Development and Comparison of Two Forms of Instruction for Training Foodservice Workers in Sanitation.* Master's thesis, Kansas State University.

School Feeding in the United States. 1947. Washington, D.C.: U.S. Department of Agriculture.

Secondary Citations. 1979. Nutrition Education and Training Project. Cambridge, Mass.: Abt Associates Inc. (December 21).

Simons, J.H. 1969. *On-the-Job Performance Following an Experimental Program for Food Service Personnel.* Iowa State University.

Southern States Work Conference on Educational Problems. 1947. *Improving Education in the Southern States: School Lunch Policies and Standards.* 1st ed. Tallahassee, Florida: The Conference.

Spears, M.C. 1977. Team Learning for Persons with Different Educational and Experience Backgrounds. *J. Am. Dietet. Assoc.* 71:146.

———. 1978. Initial Study for a Statewide Plan for Training Food Service Personnel. *School Food Service Res. Rev.* 2.

Sumbingco, S.L. 1967. *Evaluation of Programmed Textbook Presentation for Training Foodservice Employees.* Master's thesis, Kansas State University.

Swigert, E.A. 1965. *Audio-Visual Presentation of Four Motion Economy Principles for Foodservice Workers.* Master's thesis, Kansas State University.

Titles of Theses, Home Economics and Related Fields. Washington, D.C.: Agricultural Research Service, U.S. Department of Agriculture, 1955–1961.

Titles of Dissertations and Theses. Washington, D.C.: American Home Economics Association, 1962–1977.

U.S. Department of Agriculture, Food and Nutrition Service. 1971. *Guidelines for Initiating Proposals for 1971 Food Service Seminars.*

———. 1972. *The USDA Study on High School Participation in Child Nutrition Programs.*

———. 1975. *School Food Service Management Manual.* No. 1175.

———. 1977. *Principles and Practices of Sanitation and Safety in Child Nutrition Programs.* Preliminary copy (June).

———. 1979a. *National School Lunch Program, Nutritional Requirements.* Final regulations. *Federal Register* 44:48149.

———. 1979b. *Nutrition Education and Training Program.* Final regulations. *Federal Register* 44:28280.

U.S. Department of Agriculture, National Agricultural Library. 1973. *Food and Nutrition Information and Educational Materials Center Brochure.* Beltsville, Maryland.

University of Tennessee, College of Home Economics, Department of Food Science and Institution Administration. 1969. *Proceedings of Southeastern Regional Seminar for School Food Service Administrators* (June).

———. 1970. *Proceedings of Southeastern Regional Seminar for School Food Service Administrators* (June).

University of Wisconsin–Madison and Extension, College of Agricultural and Life Sciences, Department of Food Science. 1971. *Proceedings of the USDA Midwest Regional Seminar for School Food Service Supervisors and Directors: Nutrition Education and Related Management Processes* (July).

Utah State University, College of Family Life, Department of Food and Nutrition. 1971. *Proceedings of the Western Regional School Food Service Seminar: Nutrition Education in the School Food Service—Challenge, Change, and Commitment* (June).

Vaden, A.G. 1973. *Assessment of Post-Seminar Learning and of Three Methods of Contact on Innovation Efforts in Nutrition Education.* Ph.D. thesis, Kansas State University.

Wathan, G.A. 1980. *The Development of a Handbook for the School Lunchroom Employees of Cedar Rapids, Iowa.* Master's thesis, Iowa State University.

Yaussy, M.A. 1970. *An Analysis of Factors Influencing Labor Turnover Among School Food Service Personnel.* Master's thesis, University of Washington.

Young, C.S. 1966. *A Study of Non-Supervisory Employee Training in the School Lunch Programs of Massachusetts and New York.* Master's thesis, Cornell University.

5

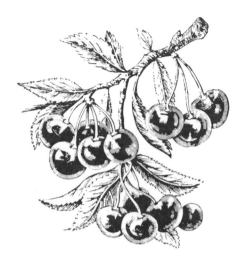

PRESCHOOL NUTRITION EDUCATION

Christine Olson and Jill Randell

INTRODUCTION

With so many approaches to preschool education, we will limit our discussion to some of the more common methods which can be applied to nutrition education curricula development or integration (Parker and Day 1977). Although each has a unique orientation, there is much overlap in theoretical foundation, goals, and methods of classroom organization. The principles underlying these approaches can be applied to the cognitive and motor skills or behavioral changes used as objectives for nutrition education at the preschool level. Many programs recognize the behavioral objective of developing appropriate food habits; others also focus on experimental techniques with cognitive and motor objectives, or on nutrition concepts, a cognitive emphasis.

In this chapter we will examine the various influences on young children's food choices. For example, parents are a major determinant in the intakes of preschool children and in their developing food habits. Nutrition education research must not overlook parents' actual and potential contributions to this process. Another influence is young children's food preferences. Nutritionally appropriate food choices can be made within these constraints, and effective programs acknowledge the common preferences of young children.

APPROACHES TO EARLY CHILDHOOD EDUCATION

The Primary Education Project is designed to "explicitly teach children the skills and concepts that underlie intelligent school performance" (Parker and Day 1977). Cumulative learning theory provides the guidelines for organizing the curriculum content. The emphasized skills are perceptual-motor, conceptual-linguistic, orienting, and attending. Learning objectives generated from task analyses are used to develop sequenced instruction activities. The classroom is organized in a way that allows the child to decide what activities to engage in and when.

The GOAL (Game-Oriented Activities for Learning) curriculum has as its primary goal "to prepare young children for effective participation in a standard school program" (Parker and Day 1977). The subgoals include cognitive development, motivation, information-processing skills, social and emotional development, and motor skill development. Learning is structured and sequenced. The teacher is provided with behavioral objectives, materials, and instructional procedures.

The Child Program's major goal is "to provide stimulation for low SES [socioeconomic status] children in order to stimulate their cognitive growth" (Parker and Day 1977). The language approach allows bilingual flexibility. The major cognitive objectives are classification and patterning, and play is emphasized to meet these objectives. Although activities are sequenced and behavioral objectives provided, they are only a "framework within which teachers may modify content and develop their own teaching strategies" (Parker and Day 1977).

The Responsive Education Program's major goals are to develop a healthy self-concept, intellectual ability, and problem-solving ability. These goals are achieved by providing a learning environment that permits the child to explore freely, select activities, and proceed at his or her own pace. The process is considered more important than the specific content. Parents are involved in many aspects of the program.

The main educational goal of the Piagetian preschool is development of the entire personality, with special emphasis on intellectual and moral autonomy. The teacher tries to understand what the child is thinking and then assists him or her in learning in the most appropriate way. Process and content are considered inseparable, with no attempt to organize or sequence the content.

The goals of the Bank Street College of Education's developmental interaction approach are "concerned with four major developmental processes [competence, individuality, socialization, and integration] and consist of supporting, stimulating, and guiding these developmental processes in the direction of selected values of optimal functioning" (Parker and Day 1977). Teaching strategies are focused on developing mutuality of trust and understanding between child and teacher; supporting a child's motivation to learn; and providing an environment to support and facilitate exploration, observation, and expression. Multiple goals are addressed in each activity.

The Montessori preschool's goal is "to provide the setting and materials through which the child, intrinsically motivated, may himself develop his intellectual, physical, and psychological abilities" (Parker and Day 1977). In a planned environment in which all materials are designed to hold the child's interest, the teacher's role is to facilitate learning and the development of concentration. The child chooses the materials to work with and the pace.

PRESCHOOLERS' FOOD PREFERENCES, CONSUMPTION, AND EATING BEHAVIOR

In contrast to past efforts in nutrition education, which have typically focused on the elementary grades, recent research and curriculum development have been directed at preschoolers' food habits and beliefs. Why has nutrition for the preschooler become a concern? How can the findings of research on preschoolers' food preferences, consumption, and eating behavior contribute to nutrition education efforts?

During the preschool years physical, emotional, and intellectual growth are especially important. Without an adequate nutritional environment, the growth of long bones may be slowed, causing permanent stunting. A hungry child, such as one who has skipped breakfast, may be apathetic and irritable. These conditions interfere with learning and are associated with iron deficiency anemia, a manifestation of malnutrition. "Early childhood educators try hard to foster intellectual curiosity, exploration and experimentation because these are the ways that young children learn; yet unresponsiveness is characteristic in malnourished children" (Foster 1972).

In addition to the effects of poor nutritional status on the child's intellectual development, nutrition education is important because food habits develop in the preschool period. These early food habits can have a lasting effect on health, considering the role of diet in tooth decay, obesity, and cardiovascular disease (Fomon 1978).

Many studies have described the eating behavior of preschool children. Early projects reported preschoolers' preferences for broiled meats, raw vegetables, and finger foods and not for combination dishes and cooked vegetables (Vance 1932, McCarthy 1935, Lamb and Ling 1946). McCarthy found that as children matured, their food preferences and aversions diminished leading to indifference toward foods.

Based on years of observing young children in nursery school, Lowenberg (1948) described preschool children's preferences for plain, unmixed, lukewarm foods and mildly flavored vegetables; dry meats were not well liked. Finger foods, a group setting, and child-sized eating utensils all enhanced the acceptance of foods.

Using multidimensional scaling techniques, Birch (1979a) found that familiarity (among three-year-olds) and sweetness (among four-year-olds) accounted for the greatest variety in choices. However, when an unfamiliar food was offered repeatedly, consumption was not affected. Birch (1979b) found a high correlation between preference and consumption and noted that three- and four-year-olds are reliable sources of information on their food preferences.

Beyer and Morris (1974), in a retrospective study of forty-four preschoolers, found eating habits fairly constant from preschool to school age. Cooked vegetables were the most disliked category (50 percent), but raw vegetables were much more acceptable. Preschoolers consumed more food as snacks relative to their total intake than did elementary school children.

These studies reflect the parents' influence on food intake. Common food preferences often result in constraining a child's dietary adequacy, because parents or other adult caretakers do not recognize their significance (for example, possible vitamin deficiencies due to inadequate intake of fruits and vegetables) or do not appreciate nutritionally acceptable alternatives among the foods a child likes (such as raw vegetables). Parents respond by forcing or bribing a child to eat, thereby fostering unacceptable behaviors, or by allowing the child to select foods at will from those available, which can lead to inappropriate intake. The parent plays a key role both by providing the food itself and by fostering appropriate or inappropriate attitudes.

Eppright et al. (1969), in surveying preschool eating behavior, found that vegetable dislikes were more closely associated with older siblings' preferences than with those of either parent. Mothers offered food as a reward 23 percent of the time, withheld it as punishment 10 percent of the time, and used it as a pacifier 29 percent of the time. While parents and children had identical aversions for one-third of the foods, McCarthy (1935) also found that older siblings had more influence on the young child's food preferences. In a study of milk consumption, preschool children were found to accept milk regardless of butterfat content or temperature (Herbert-Jackson, Cross, and Risley 1977). The negative attitudes of some older children had a greater effect on the preschoolers' reaction to a type of milk.

Bryan and Lowenberg (1958), studying the father's influence on food preferences, found that young children often liked or disliked the same vegetables as their fathers, and that foods disliked by the father were not often served by the mother.

Burt and Hertzler (1978) found that the mother and father had an equal influence on the child's food preferences. Again, the father's food likes were given high priority in planning the family menus, resulting in both parents having similar influences.

In a California study (Harper and Sanders 1975), children were given filled blue tortillas for lunch in their homes. If the mother sat down and ate similar blue tortillas, the children were much more likely to eat them than if the mothers simply offered the food.

Television advertising also has been found to influence children's food preferences. In one study the more often children were exposed to television advertisements promoting sweet foods, the more they selected these foods for snacks and meals, if given a choice (Goldberg, Gorn, and Gibson 1978).

Thus, research indicates that the characteristics of foods, including taste and familiarity, influence children's preferences. Certain foods, particularly cooked vegetables, seem to be less well liked than others. Parents, siblings, peers, and television influence children's food preferences and selections.

OVERVIEW OF PRESCHOOL NUTRITION EDUCATION PROGRAMS

Nutrition education must have as a goal the promotion of nutritional well being and good health. Nutrition education programs typically attempt to familiarize children with food and its origins, as well as to develop positive attitudes about food (Juhas 1973).

Cooking is often a part of early childhood education, but cooking is not always nutrition education. When cookies and other sweets are the focus of a cooking program, the results reinforce the child's tendency to prefer sweets. Food preparation activities, in addition to teaching positive nutrition, can support other aspects of early childhood education: math, science, language arts, art, creative expression, history, motor skills, and social-emotional development.

Nutrition education usually takes place at meals, snack time, or during carefully planned activities. Meals or snacks served family style facilitate many positive nutrition behaviors, such as tasting new foods, discussing nutrition concepts, and learning serving size (Karsch 1977).

Staff training is an important prerequisite, if a nutrition education program is to be successful (Ilg 1948, Placek 1976). Staff training must include food service workers, for they join nutrition educators in working toward the same nutrition goals (Juhas 1973). Training also is more successful when people in similar positions from a variety of organizations share ideas. Consultation with a professional nutritionist or dietitian is important not only in staff training but also in designing kitchens, developing menus and snacks, and assisting in parent education. Nutrition, use of equipment, safety procedures, and teaching techniques through role playing have been key topics in training programs (Karsch 1977).

Many curricula have provided useful information on planning and implementing food activities. Juhas (1973), Ferreira (1973), and Anselmo (1975) discuss some of the important characteristics of preschool nutrition education. While nutrition education activities that involve food can strain an already-tight budget, many programs have been successful in getting parents to contribute food, loan or donate equipment, or contribute small amounts of cash at the beginning of the school year (Placek 1976). Nutrition education activities that offer children first-hand experience, active participation, and a nonthreatening environment have been most successful (Juhas 1973, Ferreira 1973). Preparation, clean up, and serving are all part of the educational experience. Equipment should be appropriate to the child's motor skills.

Not all nutrition education activities have to involve food. Preschool teachers are successful puppet makers, storytellers, and creators of games and songs that have successfully promoted good nutrition (Smith 1976).

Other key components of preschool nutrition education are parent involvement and parent education (Placek 1976, Karsch 1977,

Ferreira 1973, Witherell 1978). A popular method of involving parents is to invite them to sample food that their children have helped to prepare. Newsletters or leaflets containing nutrition information are sometimes sent home with children (Smith 1976). Many day care and all Head Start programs emphasize parent education, and nutrition is often a topic of considerable interest to parents at workshops. Involving parents as volunteers in school nutrition activities offers several benefits in managing the activities, generating new ideas, giving parents an opportunity to learn, and providing a link between what children learn at school about nutrition and their parents' nutritional practices at home.

RESEARCH RELATED TO CHANGING THE EATING BEHAVIOR OF PRESCHOOL CHILDREN
Unevaluated Programs

The opportunities for preschool nutrition education both in and out of group settings are extensive. Some of the apparently successful, but not formally evaluated, approaches are described below.

Someone new in the classroom—a volunteer, a nutrition aide from another program, a nutrition student, or a parent—brings fresh ideas and enthusiasm to the program. Since food activities with preschoolers require close supervision, the extra hands can contribute to a successful activity and untrained volunteers can be helpful in food preparation for classroom activities, materials development, and on field trips. However, if volunteers are to teach nutrition independently, they should receive some training in nutrition and teaching techniques (Kragt 1971).

Dietetic interns were helpful in demonstrating to nursery school teachers the effectiveness of nutrition education (McDonald 1963). In a Denver Head Start program nutrition aides from the Expanded Food and Nutrition Education Program (EFNEP) taught classes to preschool children, and other aides held cooking classes for parents in their homes (Andre 1975). Coordinating parent and classroom activities proved successful in helping the children integrate what they had learned in Head Start with home life.

Other successful nutrition education efforts include sensory games and activities (Smith 1976; Frankle, Senhouse, and Cowell 1967; Marion 1978). Nutrition aides found puppets an excellent vehicle to teach nutrition to kindergarteners (Wilson, Lawroski, and Wallace 1972). A program goal was to have the children share what they had learned with their parents. Aides found parents more receptive to home visits and attributed this to the mothers' increased awareness of nutrition. Since children are exposed to many creative and entertaining advertisements that try to sell nonnutritive foods, nutrition educators are promoting healthful food habits in a similar fashion. One approach was to present a story and serve a snack to preschoolers and their parents who were shopping at a mall (Kershner and Storz 1976).

Since preschoolers love stories, the Yakima Home Economics Association developed four which promote a variety of foods, stress the importance of food for health, and inform children on how to keep food safe by proper handling (Schlick 1976).

Evaluated Programs and Approaches

The ultimate goal of nutrition education programs is to promote long-term healthful eating habits. We turn now to research projects that examine methods to improve the food habits of preschoolers. In these studies, various approaches to improving food habits have been used, including nutrition education activities, behavior modification techniques, alternative methods of serving foods, and parent involvement.

Nutrition Education Activities. Close and Sabry (1978) conducted an experiment to influence vegetable acceptance by twenty nursery school children. At-home vegetable preferences were investigated by means of questionnaires mailed to parents. Then three unfamiliar or disliked vegetables—yellow turnips, parsnips, and broccoli—were served to the children in school; their eating behavior was observed prior to an activities program. During the three-week experiment, teachers conducted various food activities in consultation with a nutritionist. After completion of the activities phase, attitudes toward the three test vegetables were again observed. In the final phase, the children's mothers were questioned about the child's current eating behavior, the parent's awareness of the food activities, and consumption of vegetables in general and of the test vegetables specifically. Children made more comments and showed more interest during food activities, particularly tasting parties, than when the food was served routinely as snacks. While the activities resulted in more children accepting the vegetables (52 percent), there were still many negative responses; 45 percent of the negative responses were to unfamiliar vegetables.

Another study measured the amount of test vegetables consumed by each child immediately after participation in a food education activity compared with that consumed at meals prior to the food education program. The education program consisted of discussion periods, dramatic exercises or games, puppets, pictures, and felt boards; real foods were used as well. The focus of each program was the vegetable served that day. After the education program, the mean intake of the four test vegetables was up 10 percent for cauliflower, 16 percent for squash, 66 percent for brussels sprouts, and 80 percent for beets. The number of children who ate some portion of vegetables increased (Harrill, Smith, and Gangever 1972).

Glaser (1957) found that after a four-month period of exposure to fruits and vegetables as part of an education program, children were more likely to accept foods that they had rejected prior to the program. The findings were based on teachers' observations and parents' comments.

Approaches Utilizing Behavior Modification. Applying behavior modification techniques to preschool children, Ireton and Guthrie (1972) attempted to increase consumption of cooked vegetables. Nineteen children, two to five years of age, from lower socioeconomic backgrounds were served five unpopular or unfamiliar vegetables—asparagus, broccoli, cauliflower, spinach, and squash—as part of five lunch menus. These menus were consistent during the two three-week experimental periods. During the first phase the method of preparation was varied (buttered, sauce, or combination); during the second phase, behavior modification techniques were used when the buttered vegetables were served. Each child received a gummed sticker upon completion of the vegetables; these stickers could be redeemed for a sweet dessert. The children also received verbal reinforcement. Although preparation had no significant effect on vegetable intake, the buttered vegetables were the preferred method (except for the sweetened squash).

In the same study token reinforcement proved a more effective means of stimulating vegetable eating behavior. During the second phase, the mean intake of vegetables was significantly higher than during the first phase. For each of the five test vegetables, a paired t-test of intakes showed a significant increase in intakes during the second phase. In addition, during the second phase 74 percent of the children were willing to taste vegetables, as compared with 32 percent during the first phase. After the study, vegetable consumption dropped but remained higher than prior to the investigation.

Hall and Holmberg (1974) investigated ways to encourage children (ages two years and seven months, and two years and eight months) to eat different kinds of foods, with no emphasis on the amount eaten. The experimental manipulations included instruction only; instruction, praise, and other rewards; praise and instruction; praise only; family style service; family style service with second helpings of foods contingent; and family style service, praise, and seconds on food contingent. The results showed individual differences, indicating the need to know what works with each child. For example, praise was most important for one child where instruction was most important for another.

Madsen et al. (1974) studied forty-six rural black children (mean age six years and two months) enrolled in a Head Start program. The amount of food eaten during breakfast was determined by weighing foods before and after the meal. In addition, observers recorded the actual amount of time spent eating. During the experimental phase, the children received verbal praise and sugar-coated cereal while eating; additional rewards were given for completing a meal. The results indicated an increase in the proportion of food consumed (from 76 percent to 93 percent) and the amount of time spent eating (from 20 percent to 33 percent) during the reinforcement (experimental) phase. Seventy-eight percent of the children increased their food consumption more than 10 percent during the reinforcement phase; four children showed increases of greater than 40 percent.

These three approaches utilizing behavior modification all succeeded to some degree but may have had negative impacts on children's nutrition. All modified attitudes or behaviors by using sweet foods (desserts and sweetened cereals) as rewards, thus incidentally reinforcing an inappropriate food behavior. Although such rewards are commonly used in behavior modification, their use is nutritionally inappropriate and cannot be condoned. Other reinforcers (praise, privileges, mutually acceptable foods) should be substituted in the future.

Parents and Adult Caregivers as Teachers and Models. Since preschool children imitate parents and other family members, a number of studies have attempted to improve children's food habits by reaching these adults. Zimmerman and Munro (1972) used behavior modification techniques with a group of Head Start mothers to improve nutrition in the home. The group was slowly introduced to a variety of nutritious foods through cooking activities. The mothers started with preferred foods and proceeded slowly, with positive reinforcement given along the way. Parents also were taught behavior modification techniques to use with their children to improve vegetable consumption. Of the twenty-two women in the group, five made dramatic changes in their meal planning at home, twelve made moderate changes, and five made very few changes.

A University of Iowa day care center found that obtaining food intake records from parents was a useful way to increase communication between parents and the center about eating problems. Nutritional benefits included planning meals to incorporate preferred foods, and increasing the children's exposure to unfamiliar foods. Nutrition education programs were also planned around the new foods (Anselmo 1975).

Highberger and Carothers (1977) studied behavioral modeling by comparing food consumption when meals were served family style (with an adult joining the children) with preplated food service (with an adult supervising). The six two-year-olds increased their consumption from 2.1 ounces of milk, 4.3 tablespoons of the main course, and 2.3 tablespoons of dessert with preplated service to 3.5 ounces of milk, 6.3 tablespoons of the main course, and 2.7 tablespoons of dessert with family style service. The adults also reinforced acceptable behavior and labeled foods, making it difficult to determine which change accounted for the increased food consumption.

Preschool Eating Patterns (PEP) involved parents in a prevention program designed to encourage weight control through the development of healthy eating habits and activity patterns in children. An interdisciplinary team led a small group meeting weekly for five weeks. The program relied on behavior modification techniques to make the desired changes; the entire family benefitted from this program. Information on the impact of this approach on children has not been reported (Smiciklas-Wright and D'Augelli 1978).

During the preschool years, children learn food habits that will sustain them through adulthood. We have reviewed some of the successful methods of teaching healthy food habits to children. Variety is considered a key to good nutritional status, and nutrition education programs have been successful in increasing the child's willingness both to taste new foods and to augment the amounts and types of foods eaten. Two other successful techniques used to supplement nutrition education for preschoolers are behavioral modeling through family meal service (adults eating with children) and behavior modification. Including parents in all aspects of the preschool program and providing them with workshops seem to help adults model nutritionally sound behaviors, learn about nutrition, and deal with the eating problems typically associated with the preschool years. These methods do not work for all children but are a good step toward improving the nutritional well-being of preschoolers.

SUMMARY AND CONCLUSIONS

Early childhood education programs have many approaches, goals, and objectives. In addition, each locality and teacher adjusts these curriculum approaches to meet particular needs. Thus, nutrition education guides and curricula must be flexible.

Since preschool children are developing food habits, nutrition goals in all curricula must include creating a positive attitude toward food, encouraging acceptance of a variety of foods, and promoting an understanding of the relationship between food and health, all leading to the development of healthful food habits.

Since many preschool teachers do not have the nutrition training to feel comfortable with nutrition activities or information, all programs must provide background information, specific guidelines for conducting the program, and references.

Nutrition activities that actively involve children can be successful in improving food habits. Structuring the educational experience or selecting the educational activity based on the child's interests and needs is a successful approach to early childhood education. Whether or not the nutrition program is integrated, the important thing is that activities are presented using a variety of modes, so that children can develop skills and learn in ways with which they are most comfortable.

Healthful food habits are encouraged by having children eat with other adults and peers. Mealtimes and snacks, with family-style service and adults eating with children, provide excellent opportunities for adults to model good eating habits, discuss nutrition with children, and use behavior modification techniques.

Parents are children's first teachers, and they continue in this role even when children begin school. Keeping parents informed about their children's nutrition education and meals or snacks served at school is important in linking school and home experiences. In addition, most parents welcome receiving nutrition information that deals with their children's food habits and preferences. Workshops, newsletters, and direct participation in the preschool program are ways to involve and inform parents. All nutrition education programs should have a parent component.

A wide variety of nutrition education curricula and resources is available for adaptation by local programs to meet specific needs. Appendix 1 provides an annotated listing of cookbooks and curricula for use in preschool nutrition education. Nevertheless, there remains a great need for research evaluating both the long-term and short-term effects of nutrition education on children during the formative preschool years.

BIBLIOGRAPHY

Andre, B. 1975. Head Start: Building Block to Better Nutrition. *School Food Service J.* 29:52.

Anselmo, S. 1975. Food Teaches! The Recipe as Lesson Plan. *Day Care and Early Educ.* (September/October): 32.

Beyer, N.R., and Morris, P.M. 1974. Food Attitudes and Snacking Patterns of Young Children. *J. Nutr. Educ.* 6:131.

Birch, L.L. 1979a. Dimensions of Preschool Children's Food Preferences. *J. Nutr. Educ.* 11:77.

————. 1979b. Preschool Children's Food Preferences and Consumption Patterns. *J. Nutr. Educ.* 11:189.

Bryan, M.S., and Lowenberg, M.E. 1958. The Father's Influence on Young Children's Food Preferences. *J. Am. Dietet. Assoc.* 34:30.

Burt, J.V., and Hertzler, A.A. 1978. Parental Influence on the Child's Food Preference. *J. Nutr. Educ.* 10:127.

Close, S.M., and Sabry, J. 1978. An Experiment to Influence Vegetable Acceptance of Nursery School Children. *J. Canadian Dietet. Assoc.* 39:221.

Eppright, E.S. et al. 1969. Eating Behavior of Preschool Children. *J. Nutr. Educ.* 1:16.

Ferreira, N. 1973. Teachers' Guide to Educational Cooking in the Nursery School. *Young Children* 24:23.

Fomon, S.J. 1978. *Nutritional Disorders of Children.* Pub. no. [HSA] 78–5104. Rockville, Maryland: U.S. Department of Health, Education, and Welfare, Public Health Service.

Foster, F. 1972. Nutrition and Educational Experience: Interrelated Variables in Children's Learning. *Young Children* 23:284.

Frankle, R.T.; Senhouse, M.F.; and Cowell, C. 1967. Project Head Start: A Challenge in Creativity in Community Nutrition. *J. Home Econ.* 59:24.

Glaser, A. 1957. Building Food Acceptances in Nursery School Children. *J. Home Econ.* 49:47.

Goldberg, M.E.; Gorn, G.J.; and Gibson, W. 1978. TV Messages for Snack and Breakfast Foods: Do They Influence Children's Preferences? *J. Consumer Res.* 5:73.

Hall, J.S., and Holmberg, M.C. 1974. The Effect of Teacher Behaviors and Food Serving Arrangements on Young Children's Eating in a Day Care Center. *Child Care Quarterly* 3:97.

Harper, L.V., and Sanders, K.M. 1975. The Effect of Adults' Eating on Young Children's Acceptance of Unfamiliar Foods. *J. Experimental Child Psych.* 20:206.

Harrill, I.; Smith, C.; and Gangever, J.A. 1972. Food Acceptance and Nutrient Intake of Preschool Children. *J. Nutr. Educ.* 4:103.

Herbert-Jackson, E.; Cross, M.Z.; and Risley, T.R. 1977. Milk Types and Temperature—What Will Young Children Drink? *J. Nutr. Educ.* 9:76.

Highberger, R., and Carothers, L. 1977. Modification of Eating Behavior of Toddlers in a Day Care Setting. *Home Ec. Res. J.* 6:48.

Ilg, F.L. 1948. The Child's Idea of What and How to Eat. *J. Amer. Dietet. Assoc.* 24:658.

Ireton, C.L., and Guthrie, H.A. 1972. Modification of Vegetable-Eating Behavior in Preschool Children. *J. Nutr. Educ.* 4:100.

Juhas, L. 1973. Nutrition Education in Day Care Programs. *J. Amer. Dietet. Assoc.* 63:134.

Karsch, B.B. 1977. Nutrition Education in Day Care. *J. Home Econ.* 69:22.

Kershner, M.H., and Storz, N.S. 1976. Nutrition Education for Preschoolers at the Shopping Mall. *J. Nutr. Educ.* 8:168.

Kositsky, V. 1977. What in the World Is Cooking in Class Today? *Young Children* 28:23.

Kragt, D. 1971. Volunteers in Nutrition Education. *J. Nutr. Educ.* 3:110.

Lamb, M.W., and Ling, B.C. 1946. An Analysis of Food Consumption and Preferences of Nursery School Children. *Child Development* 17:187.

Lowenberg, M.E. 1948. Food Preferences of Young Children. *J. Amer. Dietet. Assoc.* 24:430.

Madsen, C.H. et al. 1974. Increasing Rural Head Start Children's Consumption of Middle-Class Meals. *J. Applied Behav. Anal.* 7:257.

Marion, M.C. 1978. Touch, Taste, Smell—Feeding Nutrition into Your Program. *Day Care and Early Educ.* 5:12.

McCarthy, D. 1935. Children's Feeding Problems in Relation to the Food Aversions in the Family. *Child Development* 6:277.

McDonald, S.G. 1963. Teaching Nutrition at Nursery School Level. *Food and Nutr.* 27:672.

Parker, R., and Day, M. 1977. The Preschool in Action. In *Exploring Early Childhood Programs*. Boston, Mass.: Allyn & Bacon.

Placek, C. 1976. Kindergarten Cooks. *Day Care and Early Educ.* (September/October): 23.

Schlick, M. 1976. Kim, The Child-Approved Nutrition Teacher. *J. Home Econ.* (May): 26.

Smiciklas-Wright, H., and D'Augelli, A.R. 1978. Primary Prevention for Overweight: Preschool Eating Patterns (PEP) Program. *J. of Am. Dietet. Assoc.* 72:626.

Smith, J.M. 1976. Pathways to Preschool Nutrition Education. *Health Education* 7:14.

Vance, T.F. 1932. Food Selections of Nursery School Children. *Child Development* 3:169.

Wilson, E.H.; Lawroski, M.A.; and Wallace, A.P. 1972. Puppets Are Effective Teachers. *J. Nutr. Educ.* 4:22.

Witherell, J. 1978. From Pretzels and Potato Chips to Liver and Lettuce: A Case History. *Day Care and Early Educ.* 5:15.

Zimmerman, R.R., and Muro, N. 1972. Changing Head Start Mothers' Food Attitudes and Practices. *J. Nutr. Educ.* 4:66.

6

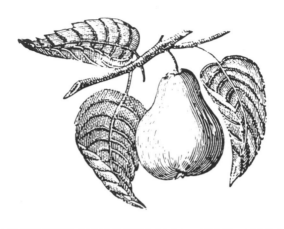

KINDERGARTEN THROUGH SIXTH GRADE NUTRITION EDUCATION

Isobel Contento

INTRODUCTION

With the passage in 1977 of PL 95–166, authorizing each state to expend $.50 per schoolchild in federal funds for "nutrition education and training" in its schools, an important step was taken to provide both food and nutrition education for the young. While activities have been carried out in both areas since the turn of the century, this legislation clearly reaffirms the importance of nutrition education and the need to integrate it with the provision of food in schools.

The federal government's action reflected the growing conviction on the part of teachers, parents, and the public during the 1970s that nutrition education was vital. This conviction was inspired in part by the realization that diet and health are related, and in part by the need of the consuming public, young and old, to find guidance in the face of a bewildering 10,000-item supermarket.

PL 95–166 was not the only response to the recent resurgence of interest in nutrition and food. Other federal offices, universities, state and local educational agencies, and health organizations, as well as the food industry, foundations, and trade associations have initiated nutrition education programs and developed a variety of educational materials, curriculum guides, and other resource materials. Teachers have included nutrition education in their curricula with increasing frequency and often voluntarily.

This review covers food and nutrition education programs conducted with, or designed for, children in kindergarten through sixth grade in the school setting. We recognize that nutrition education is being addressed by a large number of organizations and individuals, and it is impossible to review all these efforts within this chapter. Our review is limited to nutrition education programs and studies reported in the literature of the past decade and to selected curriculum guides and programs recently developed by federal, state, and local educational agencies, universities, food industries, and foundations for either local or nationwide usage.

DIETARY INTAKE AND NUTRITION STATUS: THE NEED FOR NUTRITION EDUCATION*

The nutritional status of the nation's schoolchildren has been studied extensively in several major surveys and in numerous smaller ones, which have measured the status of various age and geographic groups against various nutritional standards. Most studies measure nutrient intake as it relates to the RDAs; few studies have addressed intakes as they relate to other nutritional standards, such as the "Dietary Goals for the United States" (U.S. Senate Select Committee on Nutrition and Human Needs 1977). The actual intakes of some age groups are particularly difficult to ascertain; for instance, diets of older children eating meals and snacks away from home may be reported inaccurately. In addition to determining intakes, surveys assess nutritional status by measuring blood levels of such factors as nutrients or use anthropometric tests to analyze the long-range impact an individual's intake has on height, weight, fat stores, and so forth.

Although the following studies do not yield any definitive measures or statements, they do permit an overview of the nutritional status of children in the United States.

Ten-State Nutrition Survey (TSNS) 1968–1970

The Ten-State Nutrition Survey of 1968–1970 (U.S. Department of Health, Education, and Welfare 1972) was originally intended as a comprehensive national survey. First proposed in response to reports to Congress that nutritional deficiency diseases and clinical undernutrition existed in some parts of the country, the survey's goal was to ascertain the incidence and locations of these problems. Financial and time constraints reduced the scope of the study, limiting its findings and the projections. Using 1960 census data, researchers identified ten states' areas of lowest income. However,

*This section was contributed by Joanne Nestor.

the figures were eight years old, so some middle- and upper-income households were included in the study. Since the populations surveyed were not representative of their states or the nation, the findings could not be extrapolated; results could be used only as an indication of the status of the populations actually observed, and no others. Nevertheless, several important conclusions with implications for nutrition education were drawn:

1. A significant proportion of the low-income group was malnourished or at high risk for developing nutrition-related problems. Severity of deficiencies and nutrients which were inadequate varied with location and group.
2. Evidence of malnutrition increased as income decreased.
3. Ten- to sixteen-year-olds, particularly boys, had the most unsatisfactory nutrition status.
4. The educational level of the person buying and preparing the food was positively related to the nutritional status of children less than seventeen years old.
5. Poor food choices resulted in inadequate diets; overemphasis on red meats, relative to cheaper protein sources, was frequent.
6. A substantial number of children had calorie intakes substantially below recommended levels. An excessive number were underweight or undersize, especially in lower-income groups and states.
7. Calorie intakes varied widely, consistent with the significant numbers of both overweight and underweight individuals.
8. Poor dental care and frequency of snacking on refined carbohydrates were positively related with incidence of dental caries for most children.
9. In low-income states, school lunches provided relatively higher proportions of students' calorie, calcium, iron, and vitamin A intakes than they did in higher-income states.
10. Anemia was common in all groups. Low hemoglobin values were associated with low iron intake.
11. Low intakes and serum levels of vitamin A were found, although clinical signs were absent.
12. No major problems with vitamin C, iodine, protein or thiamin were observed.

13. Riboflavin status was poor among blacks and the young in all groups.

HANES I

The first Health and Nutrition Examination Survey (HANES I) succeeded in surveying a national sample of 20,000 from 1971 to 1975. Probabilistic design features permitted detailed analysis of preschool children, the poor, and other high-risk groups, but no cases of overt malnutrition were found. However, follicular hyperkeratosis (a vitamin A risk sign) was common among all groups, and some signs of vitamin D deficiency were found among blacks (ages one to five and eighteen to forty-four). Low iron intakes and biochemical data indicating deficiencies were found among all income and age groups.

Calorie intake was highest in above-poverty-level whites, lowest among below-poverty-level blacks. Nutrient density (per calorie) was about the same for blacks and whites, but blacks consumed fewer calories and thus had lower nutrient levels.

Rizek and Jackson (1980), using data from the National Food Consumption Surveys of 1965–1966 and 1977–1978, note that children ages six to eleven now eat 20 percent of their food away from home; in 1965 the rate was 11 percent to 15 percent, depending on age and sex. Children's consumption of separate fats and oils has decreased, as has consumption of sugar and sweets. The exception is soft drinks, which 10 percent more children now consume; girls now average 446 grams per day and boys of the same age (nine to eleven) average 413 grams. Calorie intakes have dropped.

Local Studies

The major studies, like most nutrition surveys, focused primarily or exclusively on intakes of micronutrients (vitamins and minerals), protein, and calories, compared with the levels recommended by the National Academy of Sciences Recommended Dietary Allowances (National Research Council 1974). Increasing evidence indicates that major health problems, such as heart disease, high blood pressure, cancer, diabetes, and atherosclerosis, are significantly affected by intakes of total fats, saturated fats, cholesterol, sodium (salt), sucrose, calories, and dietary fiber. Although some were not conclusive, these relationships were the focus of a set of seven "Dietary Goals for the United States" established by the U.S. Senate Select Committee on Nutrition and Human Needs (1977).

The committee recommended changes in the American diet which would help prevent or decrease the occurrence of many fatal or debilitating diseases. By comparing children's diets with these goals, poor childhood habits (for example, excess salt intake) can be identified and corrected at an early age.

The first goal, added to the December 1977 revision, was "to avoid overweight, consume only as much energy (calories) as is expended; if overweight, decrease energy intake and increase energy expenditure" (1977, p.4). The other six goals specified recommended intakes of macronutrients and sodium.

The "Bogalusa Study" of ten and eleven year olds in Bogalusa, Louisiana, found that children's mean intakes of fat and carbohydrates matched the actual intakes of the United States as a whole much more closely than they matched the levels set by the goals; intakes of sucrose and of saturated and monounsaturated fats were much higher than recommended (Foster et al. 1977). Sodium and cholesterol intakes compared favorably with the goals, but were measured in absolute rather than relative amounts; these intakes were excessive in relation to a child's body mass and calorie intake, which are smaller than those of the population as a whole. In fact, the mean caloric intake was 2,212 per day, lower than the recommended (RDA) intakes of 2,400–2,800 calories per day (depending on age and sex) for this group.

The study also found that children's snacks accounted for 34 percent of their caloric intake, including 21 percent of daily protein, 31 percent of fat, and 40 percent of carbohydrates (59 percent of sucrose). Thus, snacks, while accounting for one-third of the day's calories, supplied disproportionately small amounts of protein and large amounts of sugar and fat. Snacks provided less than one-third of the eight vitamins and minerals measured, including iron and sodium (Foster et al. 1977).

Special Groups

The population of the United States is far from homogeneous. Income and racial distinctions are not always sufficient to pinpoint groups in need, for other factors also influence food consumption patterns. The examples below demonstrate the need to recognize and address the special nutritional problems of other groups.

Native Americans and Eskimos (Alaskan Natives). The National Nutrition Policy Study (1974) found that the 800,000 Native Americans and Eskimos (Alaskan Natives) are the most impoverished and poorly nourished groups in the United States. With an average 1974 income of $1,900 per year, 40 percent of the reservation Indians fell below the poverty level, yet they paid 28 percent more for food than urban consumers. High rates of anemia were found in South Dakota, Arizona, and Alaska. White Mountain Apache children had low plasma levels of vitamin A, iron, and ascorbic acid; their incidence of anemia was two to three times that found in national surveys.

Obesity in some tribes and groups affected 60 to 90 percent of the population. The height of Eskimo children was close to the fifth percentile, but weight was close to the 50th percentile (Gonzales 1969). One-third of Navajo preschoolers in Head Start fell below the third percentile for height and tenth percentile for weight. Although Alaskan Native infants were born with lengths and weights similar to American norms, by their sixth month, lengths approached the fifth percentile. Blackfoot and Fort Belknap Indian children, however, showed growth patterns following the fiftieth percentile (Gonzales 1969).

The few limited anthropometric surveys that exist show that the average Indian preschooler is below U.S. standards for height and weight; has a high incidence of dental caries; frequently has inadequate intakes of vitamins A and C, iron, and calcium; and consumes inadequate amounts of fresh fruits and vegetables, animal proteins, and milk.

Migrants. The National Nutrition Policy Study (1974) also addressed problems of migrant workers, whose mean family income in 1971 was $1,580. Because of their low incomes, most families were eligible for federal aid programs, such as food stamps and school lunch, but frequently they were unable to take full advantage of the programs because of bureaucratic obstacles. School lunches were often not eaten because of cultural differences in food preferences, unrecognized by the lunch programs in the areas where migrants work.

Spanish-Americans. The Ten-State Nutrition Survey found that most Spanish-Americans in low-income states, particularly Mexican-Americans in Texas, had deficient intakes of vitamin A, although clinical signs of deficiency were lacking (*Nutrition Today* 1972).

Obese Children. As noted above, the first of the "Dietary Goals for the United States" is to avoid overweight. In addition to being considered a risk factor in cardiovascular disease, hypertension, atherosclerosis, diabetes, liver diseases, and so forth, being overweight is associated with poor self-image, passivity, dependency, social isolation, and real or imagined rejection (Lucas 1977).

Garn (1975) found that between 12 and 23 percent of children age six to seventeen were obese. A study by Abraham and Nordsieck (1960) found that over 80 percent of obese ten- to thirteen-year-olds were still overweight as adults. Mullins (1958) found that 30 percent of overweight adults had been overweight as children. Obesity was more common among girls of lower socioeconomic status (26 percent) than among those of higher status (3 percent) (Strunkard 1972).

Mayer (1969) observed that in most children obesity is associated with food intakes in the normal or low range and with extremely low expenditures of energy. The excess calories deposited as fat came from underexercising rather than overeating. Nutrition education programs must not assume that caloric inbalances are attributable to overeating; discussions of dieting and weight control must address exercise as well.

Conclusions

National surveys of dietary intake and nutritional status have found that most dietary deficiencies now occur only among low-income and other disadvantaged populations. Deficiency diseases, such as scurvy and rickets, are no longer problems among children.

The one exception is iron intake and iron deficiency anemias, which are prevalent among all groups. Fortification and enrichment of foods, such as bread and cereal, with nutrients once lacking in American diets has probably played a large part in eliminating these deficiencies among all but the poorest. These surveys, however, looked only at the very few nutrients with which foods are commonly fortified—a dozen of the forty nutrients known to be required. "Current research suggests that a variety of essential but poorly studied nutrients—zinc, magnesium, and vitamin E, for example—may in fact be significant for some fraction of the population" (*Nutrition Today,* 1972, p. 10). Since these nutrients are not used to fortify or enrich refined foods, we must not take the available research as proof that deficiencies are not a problem. Rather, this evidence points to the need to reduce the intake of refined foods in favor of less processed foods, which usually contain greater amounts of the nutrients we know less about.

Most current nutrition-related health problems relate to dietary excesses and imbalances rather than deficiencies. Recent dietary goals and recommendations focus on the reduction of factors known to have adverse effects on health when consumed in excess, such as sugar, salt, calories, and saturated fats. Available evidence indicates that children are forming lifelong inappropriate dietary habits in these areas.

Finally, children with special economic, cultural, and behavioral needs must not be overlooked. Varying food preferences, beliefs, attitudes, and purchasing power all influence intake and status. Nutrition education programs must adapt their messages and techniques to their audiences. The best technique, project, or curriculum is that which is tailored to the special needs of the particular group.

CONTEXT AND THEORETICAL REVIEW

Nutrition education has been defined as "the process which enables individuals to gain understanding and skills necessary to promote and protect their nutritional well-being through their food choices" (Ullrich 1979). The ultimate aim is a general improvement of nutritional status through improved food intake. This in turn depends on participation in eating events; participation is influenced by biological needs and a variety of other factors, such as nutrition knowledge, food values, economic resources, and eating opportunities. Today's schools are paying attention to all these factors.

Nutrition Knowledge and Food Values: The Content of Nutrition Education

While improved nutritional status has remained a national goal over the years, the knowledge, skills, and attitudes needed to meet this goal have changed. At the turn of the century, when poverty and malnutrition were rampant, this goal was expressed as a need to upgrade the nutritional quality of the diet by supplementing it with highly nutritious foods, so that children could benefit from schooling and grow into adults who would be productive workers. People were urged to add more calories and protein foods to their diets. Indeed, in 1908 Dr. Emerson of Boston developed a "nutrition class method" for encouraging underweight children to compete with each other in weight gains (Whitehead 1957). The results were so spectacular that he was invited all over the country to train people in his weight gain method. With the discovery during the 1930s and 1940s of the importance of vitamins and minerals, education came to involve teaching children to add "protective" foods —fruit and vegetables—as well as calories and protein to their diets.

Today, however, the average American eats twice as much protein as needed, and deficiencies of the major vitamins and minerals are not widespread. Thirty percent of the population is overweight and must avoid not deficiencies in the major nutrients, but such apparently nutrition-related degenerative illnesses as heart disease, diabetes, cancer, hypertension, and possibly deficiencies in the trace nutrients.

Thus, earlier in this century, a nutritionally sound diet required the individual to learn which foods provided adequate protein and protective substances—vitamins and minerals—in order to be certain to include these in the diet, and to try a number of nutritious foods which may have been new or unfamiliar.

In contrast with yesterday's need to include foods high in protein, vitamins, and minerals, today's learner must be informed to select wisely from the vast array of foods available. The individual must discriminate about dietary advice that comes, sought and unsought, from a variety of equally reliable sources and must develop food selection attitudes and behaviors conducive to long-term health. As one researcher said, "In the past, the message was, in essence, to eat more of everything. Now we are faced with the more difficult problem of teaching the public to be more discriminating. Increasingly, the message will be to eat less" (Hegsted 1979).

Nutrition education has drawn largely from biochemistry in attempting to meet the goal of a healthy population. As a consequence, nutrition educators generally have focused on teaching children how to apply nutrition science principles (that is, food-grouping systems and nutrients) to food selection (Picardi and Pariser 1975, Robinson 1976). Traditionally, such approaches have not always taken into account rapid changes in the food supply and the consequent changing educational needs of children, nor have they provided the link between acquired knowledge and behavioral change. Therefore, nutrition educators need to develop curricula and programs that offer informative activities which promote eating habits conducive to long-term health—in the context of the current and anticipated American food supply.

Nutrition Knowledge and Food Values: The Process of Nutrition Education

Improvement of nutritional status depends not only on what is taught about foods and nutrition, but on how it is taught. Obviously, it is good for people to "know" nutrition; it is even better if they develop desirable eating behavior. Nutrition education attempts to produce both effects.

Emerson's "class method" was highly successful in bringing about weight gains in underweight children and was emulated throughout the country. Dr. Lydia Roberts in 1917 used both the "individual method" and the "class method" with children in a clinic setting in Chicago (Roberts 1927). Advanced nutrition students from the University of Chicago assisted in the clinic and received training in methods of improving child nutrition. At the same time, Mary Swartz Rose of Teachers College, Columbia University, and Mary Harper, nutritionist for the New York Association for Improving the Conditions of the Poor, developed similar programs in New York City (Whitehead 1957, Roberts 1927). Both Roberts, who came into the field as an experienced teacher, and Rose, who worked in a teacher's college, recognized that nutrition education could be more effective in a school setting than in clinics. Every child could be reached through the public schools, not just the "under par." As early as 1913, other educators began to see opportunities for nutrition education within school programs (Langworthy 1913, Legget 1913, Creswell 1913). Although the goal of nutrition education was still improvement of child nutrition, the emphasis shifted to the "teaching" of nutrition.

As with other subjects, over the years the teaching of nutrition has drawn from the education theories and practices currently in vogue. In the early 1900s Dewey and others rejected the rote learning approach of an earlier era and emphasized the importance of the learner and the real world context in which learning took place. An integrated approach was advocated, combining the teaching of nutrition with science lessons, number work, spelling, cooking lessons, work in school gardens, and the like. One researcher already had considered school lunch programs (offered in forty-one cities at the time) as "a working laboratory for giving instruction concerning the pure food movement, food costs, food values, and the relation of food to working efficiency" (Langworthy 1913).

Classroom instruction also was influenced by Dewey's emphasis on the importance of thinking in experience and on education for a democracy as education in thinking. "Learning by doing" and problem solving rather than rote learning became the core of educational practice. Rose, for example, believed that the appropriate tool for teaching nutrition was food, so each lesson was built around a specific food found regularly in the children's diets. Since she agreed that children learn by doing, activities were part of each class, and children were responsible for conducting the activities. The nutrition subject matter, Rose urged, must be graded to take into account the experience and understanding of the students, facts must relate to individual and community needs, and parents must be involved (Rose 1932). The ultimate goal of nutrition education was to help the child "deal wisely with his appetite and make habitually profitable selections of food for himself" (Eagles, Pye, and Taylor 1979).

Variations on the problem-solving approach, with its emphasis on reasoning skills, have been used over the years. Activity-oriented and "discovery learning" strategies have been used widely. Most of nutrition education in school in the 1960s and early 1970s, however, still relied rather heavily on strategies best described as information transmission methods ultimately derived from behaviorist theories. An analysis of the major kindergarten through grade twelve curriculum guides used in 1976, for example, showed that the suggested learning activities were strongly teacher-dominated, and that active student participation was found only in a little over half of them (Cooper and Go 1976). Furthermore, the objectives of teaching units were primarily in the cognitive domain, with most at the lower levels of the cognitive taxonomy, requiring only knowledge and comprehension.

Fortunately, some nutrition educators agreed with Bosley, who in 1946 noted: "Nutritionists and educators should not lose sight of the real reason for nutrition education in their eagerness to disseminate information. The aim of nutrition education is a simple one: to establish good habits which will result in intelligent food selection, day by day, throughout life" (Bosley 1947).

Through the years, many nutrition educators have been concerned with encouraging appropriate eating behavior and have attempted to measure behavioral outcomes. McKenzie and Mumford concluded from their review of forty papers that "The success or failure of an educational programme depends on the methods used, the personalities involved, and the circumstances prevailing in the area at that time" (1965). They were not in a position to isolate these factors but urged that "social scientists and nutritionists work in close cooperation to establish a satisfactory and simple methodology and to encourage the use of evaluation as an integral part of any programme they design" (1965). After reviewing 269 items published between 1900 and 1970, Whitehead noted that much of nutrition education was directed "toward the purpose of disseminating nutrition information rather than toward the purpose of improving dietary habits" (1970). From those studies which did attempt to bring about changes in eating patterns, she concluded that "problem solving is an effective way to influence what people do about their dietary intakes and their food supply" (1970). People need to be involved in the planning, development, and evaluation of nutrition education, although "such education should be supervised by adequately prepared nutrition educators"

(1970). Effective nutrition education should actively involve learners in the process.

In the past decade there has been an increasing insistence that nutrition education efforts be evaluated not just on gains in nutrition knowledge but also on changes in eating behavior. Appropriate knowledge does not automatically result in appropriate behavior, nor can we depend on the assumption that knowledge influences attitudes, which in turn influence behavior. Thus, if our goal is to bring about desirable eating behavior, we must use behavioral measures to evaluate our success. Given the complex relationship among knowledge, attitudes, and behavior (Zimbardo, Ebbeson, and Maslich 1979; Swanson 1972), where in some situations changed behaviors seem to result from changed attitudes and in others changed attitudes result from changed behaviors, any measures used to evaluate success in influencing eating behavior must be interpreted and extrapolated with care.

Economic Resources and Eating Options: School Meals

The nation's school feeding programs began in the early 1900s. The early urban school breakfast and penny lunch programs were funded and operated mainly by various women's groups, such as the General Federation of Women's Clubs, the National Council of Jewish Women, and the National Congress of Mothers (Reese 1980). Unlike the older philanthropic organizations, such as the Salvation Army, these women's groups favored state funding, provision, and control. By World War I about one hundred cities had meal programs of some sort controlled by voluntary groups. These programs varied widely and reached only a small proportion of elementary school children. Federal and state extension workers helped set up school lunch programs in the rural areas.

In 1946 the National School Lunch Act was passed. It had evolved during the 1930s and early 1940s when, although the youth of the nation faced malnutrition, vast quantities of surplus food were accumulating because Americans could not afford to buy. The act was designed "as a measure to safeguard the health and well-being of the Nation's Children and to increase the market for nutritious Agricultural Commodities" (Martin 1978, Whitehead

1957). Roberts believed that the act should be "an educational measure as well as one for safeguarding the health of pupils" (1927). In fact the authors of the original bill had proposed that $18 million be included annually for nutrition education and training; that component, however, was eliminated in the political battles that followed. The Child Nutrition Act, which in 1966 added a number of food programs, such as the breakfast and free milk programs, had inserted a nutrition education component in 1970. However, not until the 1977 amendments to the National School Lunch Act was a comprehensive component finally enacted. While some have viewed school meals as a welfare program, others as a service, and still others as a way to use up excess food commodities, these recent legislative actions clearly establish the importance of school meals as an educational tool.

Economic Resources and Eating Options: Political Relationship with Community Services

"Grants for Demonstration Projects to Improve School Nutrition and Health Services for Children from Low-Income Families" was enacted as an amendment to Title VIII of the 1965 Elementary and Secondary Education Act (ESEA), under Section 808 in PL 91-230, in April 1970. Section 808, a national competitive program under which the U.S. Office of Education made direct grants to local educational agencies (LEAs), sought to demonstrate how LEAs could exercise leadership in linking eligible children and their families to food and health services in their communities.

In 1976 Congress consolidated several former programs, including Section 808, into ESEA Title IV-C. The purposes of Title IV-C are quite broad: to assist in the provision of vitally needed educational services, to stimulate the development of exemplary elementary and secondary programs to serve as models to others, and to support demonstration projects designed to improve nutrition and health services in public and private schools with high concentrations of children from low-income families. There is no mandate that a state must solicit and fund health and nutrition projects specifically (Powers 1978).

Summary

The content of nutrition education should help develop in youngsters food behavior conducive to long-term health. The process of nutrition education should bring about not only gains in knowledge, but the development of desirable attitudes and food behavior. Nutrition education in the classroom, our next section, should be integrated with the lunchroom experience and with community resources.

NUTRITION EDUCATION STUDIES

In December 1969 the "White House Conference on Food, Nutrition, and Health" called for a renewed interest in nutrition education in the schools. Called in part because of the hunger and malnutrition in America that had been brought to national attention, this conference reemphasized some of the features of the 1966 Child Nutrition Act, which had not only required lunch and breakfast programs in the schools but had also provided for nutrition education for school personnel. The "Panel on Nutrition Teaching and Education" recommended a series of concepts taught in the classroom but also urged the use of school cafeterias as "laboratories for applying nutrition principles taught in classrooms" (White House Conference on Food, Nutrition, and Health 1970).

Six years later, to assess the follow-up action on the White House nutrition education recommendations, the National Nutrition Education Clearing House (NNECH) surveyed all fifty states and the District of Columbia (Johnson and Butler 1975). Of forty-two respondents, ten states had legislated policy concerning nutrition education; many others were formulating programs. Twenty-three states had curriculum guides that included nutrition, and thirty-one had a state director for nutrition education. Nutrition education was implemented through a range of disciplines and methods.

A comprehensive study done at about the same time (1975) by the Education Commission of the States indicated very similar findings. Thirty-one of the fifty responding states reported either having or planning to have an office responsible for nutrition education. About 30 percent of the state education agencies (SEAs) and about 40 percent of the local education agencies (LEAs) responding had projects or programs using federal, state, local, or private funds. More than 75 percent of the states, about 40 percent of the responding LEAs, and 17 percent of the responding private schools sponsored activities in nutrition education for school food service personnel. Nutrition education was taking place in the nation's schools, but it was largely on a voluntary basis. Nutrition educaton was ranked low in priority in comparison to other health education areas by SEAs, LEAs, and private schools, and the low level of interest on the part of school superintendents was reflected in the small proportion of budgets allocated to nutrition education. Nevertheless, the survey noted that where taught, nutrition education was becoming a component of the integrated curriculum movements occurring in public and private schools throughout the nation.

To find out how much time was spent on nutrition in the elementary classroom, Cook, Eiler, and Kaminaka surveyed 2,160 elementary teachers in New Jersey and New York. Three-fourths of the respondents said they had taught foods or nutrition in their classrooms in the previous year, averaging 9.7 hours of class time during the year, with somewhat more time for kindergarten through third grade than for grades four through six. Most of the teachers thought nutrition was "important" but felt it should be taught by someone else at some other grade level.

In a report on Title IV-C programs, Powers (1978) noted that Section 808 had funded a total of twenty-three projects in twenty-one states between 1970 and 1976. Each of these was funded for one to three years, and altogether an estimated 32,600 children were served. In FY 1977, eighteen states reported approving funds for forty health and nutrition education projects.

These surveys and others demonstrate that interest in and implementation of nutrition education programs have both increased enormously in the past decade and especially in the past five years.

Nutrition Education Reported in the Literature

During the past ten years, the variety and number of nutrition education activities in the schools have increased to avalanche proportions. Many are conducted voluntarily by the classroom teacher or the food service manager and are not reported anywhere. Hundreds of other efforts are funded by mini-grants awarded by a variety of agencies and organizations. They are no doubt detailed in reports to their funding sources, but only a few of these activities are reported in the literature. Thus, articles appearing in the literature, our only easily available sources of information on such programs, represent only a fraction of the nutrition education going on in the United States today.

We applied several criteria in selecting reports for review. First, the nutrition education reported had to represent a program or series of coordinated food and nutrition education events; single events were excluded. Second, the program had to have been carried out in the past decade. Third, the report could not be a master's or doctoral thesis. Fourth, the article had to describe some method used to evaluate the nutrition education effort. We decided to include studies in which success was assessed subjectively by those involved, such as food service workers, teachers, students, or parents, as well as those in which success was measured objectively by one or more criteria. Of the sixty or so articles that seemed to fit these criteria based on either their titles or their abstracts, only twenty-two met the criteria upon closer examination; the remainder turned out to be suggestions for improving nutrition education or encouraging reduction of school plate waste. While extremely important to practitioners, such articles did not concern evaluated programs.

Studies Reporting Subjective Assessments. Studies using subjective judgments for evaluating nutrition education were included for two reasons. First, these studies provide examples of the kinds of educational activities that go on in real teaching environments (as opposed to situations in which research studies are being conducted, which inevitably alter the teaching environment). Second, there is a lack of well-tested, appropriate methodologies for assessing the effects of nutrition education, especially behavioral effects.

Nine studies are included in this group. Most were reported in the last five years, and they are described chronologically.

Dobbins (1971) reported on a number of programs carried out in Oklahoma City. Teachers in elementary schools were provided inservice training. Joint efforts by food service personnel and by teachers at Broken Arrow Elementary School were reported as having "increased participation in the school feeding programs by a little over 25% and decreased plate waste almost 50%" (Dobbins 1971). However, no data were presented to substantiate this statement, and the report was otherwise qualitative in its description. Parents became so interested in the programs that special classes were organized for them.

George (1971) embarked on a three-week study with his sixth graders. Students recorded their daily meals and worked with the head cook of their rural school to plan a week of lunches for the school lunch program. This activity was accompanied by filmstrips, charts, and discussions about balanced meals. Students enacted skits to publicize their planned menus to the other grades. The students' food diaries and a short test were used to evaluate the results, which were described as "outstanding," and enthusiasm was high among both students and parents.

Zumsteg (1976) described the integrated food and nutrition education efforts in a Minnesota school district of 33,000 students. One part of the program consisted of setting up "tasting tables" where taste-size portions of any new food, especially vegetables, were served. Children who finished the first portion could return for more. In another part of the program the cook-managers in the schools demonstrated food preparation and visited classrooms to talk about food and nutrition. The staff found that "when children recognize a food they have eaten before in some form, they tend to accept it more easily" (Zumsteg 1976). A third part consisted of providing students with opportunities in the classroom to prepare parts of the school lunch, such as soups, with vegetables supplied by the cafeteria. School personnel, as well as the children, were reported to be very "enthusiastic" about the programs and the parents "very positive." Each term, parents received newsletters and fliers containing news about the program, as well as nutrition and food information.

In 1976 the Edmond, Oklahoma, school food service directors and teachers designed a nine-lesson nutrition education program conducted in the school's cafeteria. The programs consisted of watching filmstrips, playing games, preparing and tasting food, and taking home food samples along with snack recipes for the children's parents. Teachers reported that "more children were eating school lunches," and "discussing the food groups system at lunch." Parents found that "their children were more willing to try new and different foods at home and school," students were discussing the Basic Four at home, and "many children began eating breakfast" ("Nutrition Education Is as Easy as 1, 2, . . . 9" 1976).

By letting students plan their own menus, one school successfully integrated nutrition education in the classroom with school lunch, with beneficial results in both settings. The program's goals were student involvement, nutritious meals, and clean plates. Six-, seven-, and eight-year-olds were provided food and nutrition information while designing menus for school lunch. Garbage cans, labeled according to the Basic Four, were placed in the lunchroom, and at the end of each lunch period, garbage bags were weighed in both English and metric units; milk was measured in quarts and liters. Students recorded the amounts of uneaten food each day on a large chart near the school entrance. "Close to empty" garbage cans formed one measure of success of the program; the enthusiasm of those involved was another (Halfacre 1977).

DeZeeuw described the use of student advisory councils (SACs) to encourage nutrition education in the elementary schools. Two schools in South Carolina, for example, had some thirty students involved in each of their SACs. These students planned menus and participated in special projects, such as food habit surveys, plate waste studies, and puppet shows. As a result of such activities, plate waste was reduced and "more children are eating a larger variety of foods and liking the foods they had not tried before" (1979).

One school district of 24,000 students used a comprehensive team approach involving food service professionals, teachers in all subject areas, and administrators (King 1979). In the elementary schools nutrition was integrated into the teaching of other subjects. For example, a "grocery store center" was used to teach the Basic Four and math. One cafeteria manager worked with sixth graders in planning, cost accounting, and merchandising the menus for greater student participation. Nutrition education thus assisted in the development of basic skills. Teachers also reported that "students can become concerned about and self-directed in their food choices with significant carry over into their homes" (King 1979).

Theater was used in one elementary school to teach about vegetables ("Vegetables on Parade" 1979). A package developed by the Potato Board included a script for a play, entitled "Vegetable

Parade," lesson plans for teachers, and suggested student activities for classrooms and school cafeterias. While preparing for the performance, students tasted the vegetables and learned about their nutritional value. The play was followed by a tasting party at which guests and participants sampled and enjoyed various kinds of vegetables prepared by the students. Evaluations by teachers who used this program were described as follows: "Ninety-one percent felt students learned to identify a wide variety of vegetables; 93% felt the program created a positive student attitude toward vegetables with specific vitamins and minerals; and 100% felt that students learned that vegetables should be eaten every day" ("Vegetables on Parade" 1979, p.50). No data were presented to substantiate these conclusions.

Parents took the initiative to increase nutrition education in one New York City school (Kamhi 1980), and the effort eventually involved all segments of the school community. Drawing upon the U.S. Dietary Goals as a conceptual framework and using both classrooms and the school cafeteria as learning laboratories, the program emphasized minimally processed foods that were low in added fat, sugar, and salt. A food grouping system, called the Perfect Plate, was devised, in which a circle consisted of three wedges —the largest for grains, the second for fruits and vegetables, and the third for protein foods—with a narrow sliver for fats. The foods and drinks used in classroom activities and parties also were changed to conform to the Dietary Goals. Both parents and teachers, "observing the healthy changes in the children's eating habits," judged the program successful (Kamhi 1980). Children also compiled a notebook of comments on how the program affected them.

Studies Reporting Objective Assessments. We found only twelve studies conducted in the past decade reporting objective assessments of the effects of nutrition education on children in kindergarten through sixth grade. The evaluation measures used were knowledge gained, attitudes or preferences changed, or desirable behavior developed. Several reports concerned validation studies of curricula designed for wide usage. These studies are included in the discussions of specific curricula.

In 1970 Lovett, Barker, and Marcus reported on a study designed to determine the effectiveness of the Dairy Council of California's

Big Ideas program for second graders. The sample consisted of 1,720 students in 71 schools in Los Angeles. The students were divided into three groups: the experimental group, whose teachers were trained by Dairy Council personnel and equipped with its materials; the semicontrol group, whose teachers were supplied with the same materials and with general objectives derived from California state health textbooks; and a control group, whose teachers were supplied only with the general objectives. Classes were pretested in nutrition knowledge and balanced meal selection, taught a nutrition course averaging one hour per day for three weeks, and posttested.

Although no statistical tests were reported, classes taught by trained teachers using supplied materials (the experimental group) showed a 360 percent improvement in identifying the Basic Four; the semicontrol and control groups showed improvements of 51 percent and 76 percent, respectively. Seventy-five percent of the experimental group could identify all four food groups and showed a 151 percent increase from pre- to post-test in the ability to select a balanced breakfast, lunch, and dinner, satisfactorily choosing one and one-third meals instead of less than one complete meal. The semicontrol and control groups showed an improvement of 39 percent and 22 percent, respectively. Thus, the students who were taught nutrition by trained teachers, using prepared materials, showed improvement in nutrition knowledge and the ability to select balanced meals; behavioral changes were not reported.

Baker (1972) reported on a study undertaken in an Iowa county, where a previous survey had shown that students had low intakes of calcium, iron, and vitamins A and C. Approximately 200 fourth and fifth graders participated in the study; about half were in classes that served as the experimental group. The outcomes were evaluated in terms of physical, attitudinal, and dietary changes, as well as nutrition knowledge and scholastic achievement scores.

The objectives were for children to (1) learn how to formulate a concept of health involving optimum well-being, (2) comprehend the dependence of health on food, (3) improve food habits if needed, and (4) recognize that diet interacts with many factors to affect health. The learning experiences were organized into thirteen thirty-minute lessons given daily, plus two follow-up lessons. They were taught by the researcher, usually during the health or science periods. Lesson plans were identical for the two grades and were highly activity-oriented. Children made growth charts, observed cells under a microscope, fingered milk ash, bent a decalcified bone, tested foods for fat and starch, and observed an animal-feeding demonstration.

The nutrition test consisted of multiple-choice test items derived from the stated behavioral objectives. The same test was given before and after the three-week nutrition education program. Two-hour dietary recalls and one twenty-four-hour dietary record were obtained for each child before and after the nutrition unit. A seven-point hedonic scale of facial expressions was used to rate liking of nine vegetables before and after the program. Scores on the Iowa Every Pupil Test of Basic Skills, administered several months before and again several months after the program, were obtained from school records.

Baker found that between the pre- and post-testing periods, test scores of the experimental group improved significantly more (p < .01) than did those of the control group. No significant changes attributable to the nutrition education unit were found for the nutritive and caloric values of children's diets; the scores on scholastic achievement tests; children's vegetable preferences; or changes in height, weight, skinfold thickness, or arm and leg girths. Baker reported that although a number of activities assisted children in attaining the stated objectives, those requiring children to classify foods according to their caloric and nutritive values were not among them. Two and one-half years later, parents were questioned about factors influencing their children's diets during the period of the nutrition survey and the nutrition education program. Parents cited influences that were unrelated to either event, such as "TV and radio ads" and "changes in school lunches and snacks."

Boysen and Ahrens (1972) used knowledge tests, a lunch survey, and a parent questionnaire to measure the results of a four-week nutrition education program for second graders. Fifty-nine students participated in the study, with thirty in one class serving as the experimental subjects and twenty-nine in another class serving as controls. The goals of the program were to foster an awareness of the need for good food and an understanding of and ability to use the Basic Four grouping system to improve food habits.

Presented in thirty-minute daily segments during the four weeks, the program consisted of student-oriented activities. Students played games to practice classification of foods into the four groups and to plan well-balanced breakfasts and lunches. The students checked their own diets for adequacy in terms of the food groups and held a "good nutrition" party.

Performance on the pre- and post-tests of nutrition knowledge was measured in terms of the percent of right answers. Students in the experimental group improved their test scores more than students in the control group. Statistical tests of significance were not given.

For two weeks before and two weeks after the program, both classes had their lunches evaluated for content before eating and for waste after eating. The researchers found that among both groups the quality of lunches brought from home was poor and that the waste of certain items was high in both home and school lunches. One-fourth of the students drank no milk with lunch, 50 percent to 60 percent brought no fruit, and 90 to 95 percent no vegetables, although 95 percent brought cookies or highly salted snacks in addition to their sandwiches. Food item waste was measured in terms of the proportion of each individual portion left uneaten. Those items wasted most were fruit and milk from home, and vegetables, salad, and milk from school meals. The experimental group showed a slight improvement in their willingness to try milk, but the differences between the groups were not substantial. Of the twenty-two parents responding to a questionnaire, half said they felt their child's eating habits had changed for the better; but only the parents of the experimental groups were surveyed, and the comments reported were subjective and general. This short program, like that conducted by Head (1974), was reported as improving the students' nutrition knowledge, but not their eating habits.

Bell and Lamb (1973) used changes in cognitive learning and dietary behavior to measure the effects of a six-week nutrition instruction module administered to approximately 1,500 fifth graders in 33 schools. Students were randomly divided into control and experimental groups by classroom.

The module used was the Big Ideas program designed by Dairy Council, Inc. Its emphasis was on food classification, balanced meals, and nutritional analysis of foods from the Basic Four. Learning experiences included games, discussions, reports, menu planning, tasting parties, and an animal-feeding experiment.

The nutrition test was a twenty-five-item objective test of students' knowledge, comprehension, and application; the same test was used for the pre- , post- , and retention tests. The results showed that the experimental groups had a significantly higher posttest mean score than the control group at the 0.001 level. The mean increase in the experimental group posttest scores was 31 percent, and in the control groups, 8 percent. These differences were maintained in the retention test given six weeks later.

For five consecutive days before and after the module, dietary changes were assessed by changes in vegetable and milk consumption, which were problem areas for the children. Unconsumed vegetables were measured on a group basis from the amount served and from plate waste; leftover milk portions were pooled and measured. Vegetable consumption increases were statistically significant in the experimental groups compared with the control groups, but the change was small (6.1 percent versus 0 percent). The gain in milk consumption in the experimental groups was not significantly greater than in the control groups, and both were small (8.0 percent and 3.9 percent).

Head (1974) reported on a five-month nutrition education program for fifth, seventh, and tenth graders which was evaluated on cognitive, affective, and behavioral measures. Part of an Office of Economic Opportunity–funded comprehensive survey of the School Lunch Program in North Carolina, the study was stimulated by a previous survey of nutritional status. The objectives were to change food habits or acceptability of foods served in the program. Nutrition education was introduced in two elementary, two junior high, and two high schools. Control data were obtained from five matched schools in the same geographic area. In each experimental school matched classes served as within-school controls for the two or more nutrition education classes in the school. Nutrition education was given to four fifth grade, four seventh grade, and four tenth grade classes, with an average class size of twenty-six; some 4,700 students were included in both the experimental and the control groups.

In the fifth grade classes teachers integrated nutrition into other courses. Scrapbooks, skits, field trips, food preparation, and tasting parties were among the techniques used. In the seventh grade the health courses incorporated nutrition; in the tenth grade nutrition was integrated with biology.

Researchers administered the nutrition test to fifth grade students orally. Food acceptability was determined by presenting students with the daily menu on a card which had space to check attitudes toward each food on a five-point scale. Food consumption behavior was evaluated by means of plate waste studies and three-day dietary records.

Significant differences (p = 0.05) were found between the post-test scores of the nutrition education and control classes for all the fifth grade groups and for one seventh grade group. Dietary records showed that seventh graders receiving nutrition education improved their diets (p = 0.05) more than control classes, but fifth graders did not. There was a significant difference (p = 0.05) in plate waste between experimental and control fifth grade groups, but not in other groups. Waste of foods high in vitamins, minerals, and protein decreased considerably. Acceptability ratings of school-served food increased among fifth grade experimental groups more than among other groups. However, among none of the groups was the change in acceptability significant. Additional data indicated among fifth graders a significant correlation between the acceptability rating assigned to a food and the quantity of that food consumed.

This rather complex study thus demonstrated that among fifth graders nutrition knowledge increased, plate waste decreased significantly, and food acceptability increased slightly. Head noted that "improvement in diets of fifth grade nutrition education groups was probably masked by the marked improvements in the diets of both experimental and control groups" (1974). One group of seventh graders improved their knowledge of nutrition; their three-day dietary records also reflected an improvement in their diets. The tenth graders did not improve in any category. Thus the amount of change resulting from nutrition education with the instructional methods used in this study "decreased progressively at higher grade levels."

Jenkins, Stumo, and Voichick (1975) evaluated the effects of the nutrition education program "Mulligan Stew" on 140 fourth graders in four schools in two cities. They measured changes in nutrition knowledge and dietary intake by using three-day food records. Four classes, taught by classroom teachers, served as the experimental group and two as the control group. The program consisted of a series of six films and supplementary learning materials; the films were shown at weekly intervals, with thirty minutes of supplementary activity scheduled after each film. The major source of supplementary material was a "Mulligan Stew" workbook in comic book format.

The nutrition knowledge test consisted of thirty-seven multiple choice or fill-in questions and was administered one week before and one week after viewing the complete film series. Similarly, three-day records of food intake were completed one week before and one week after. The experimental classes as a whole scored significantly higher on the posttest than did the control groups (p < .01). In general, food records indicated that diets contained smaller amounts of each of the five nutrients calculated after the program than before; however, the energy value of the diet did not change. In one city there was no difference in the diet changes between experimental and control classes. In the other city the experimental groups' diets improved slightly or did not change, while those of the controls showed decreases in nutrient intake. Children in groups showing dietary improvement also showed the largest increase in nutrition knowledge.

Wang and Dwyer (1975) also used the "Mulligan Stew" nutrition education program with fifty-six fourth and sixth graders. The researchers were interested in whether cognitive and behavioral changes could be encouraged with a culturally distinct group (American-Chinese children) by using the film series supplemented with culture-specific instruction. Three classes participated in the study: in one, only the six "Mulligan Stew" films were shown weekly, each lasting thirty minutes; in the second class, thirty minutes of culture-specific instructions were given, as well as the films; and the third class received thirty minutes per week of only culture-specific instruction.

The objective of the film series is to teach children of low-income families good nutrition by repeatedly illustrating food selection based on the Basic Four. In this study the nonfilm instruction was specifically designed to associate Chinese foods and cultural concepts with the Basic Four. Two techniques, a previously designed and tested questionnaire and a food feast, were used to evaluate the efficacy of the three variations in instructional method. The questionnaire had three sections: the first assessed the children's food-related activities, such as grocery shopping or making breakfast; the second recorded children's meal and snack selections for one day; the third tested nutrition knowledge. The questionnaire was modified from its original form for Chinese food habits and was given in both English and Chinese. A second instrument was administered during a food feast, at which children could choose from a number of Chinese and American snack foods (some of which fitted into the Basic Four). The children recorded their choices on the back of the questionnaire.

On the nutrition knowledge subtest, differences between pre- and post-test scores were significant only for children who had been exposed to culture-specific instruction, with or without the film series. Only the children exposed to both films and classroom instruction scored significantly higher in the meal selection section of the questionnaire. Those exposed only to the films scored significantly lower in the food feast than did the other two groups. The researchers noted that the culture of the Chinese-Americans studied differed greatly from the culture portrayed in the film series; this perhaps accounted for the observed differences in efficacy of the culture-specific instruction and of the films when shown alone.

In summary, this study showed that both a significant increase in knowledge of nutrition and improved food selection ability were related to the provision of culture-specific classroom instruction. The implication is that, to be effective, the orientation and content of nutrition education materials must be culturally relevant to the learner.

With fifth graders, Meyers and Jansen (1977) tested the effectiveness of a nutrition education unit using a nutrient approach. The basic tool was a "nutrient abacus" or nutri-planner, which could be used to evaluate and plan school lunches by considering content of calories and eight nutrients. Rows of beads, representing the different nutrients, could be added to reach the school lunch nutrient standard of one-third of the RDAs.

By integrating classroom learning with the school lunch program, the study was designed not only to provide children with basic nutrition knowledge but also to acquaint them with some of the dietary problems associated with today's eating patterns. Five fifth grade classes, containing ninety-four students, participated in the study. Four classes comprised the experimental group, and the fifth class was the control group. Classroom teachers (provided with three inservice sessions) taught the unit for forty minutes per day for three weeks. The unit was planned to coincide with a unit on cells in the science syllabus. Cartoon characters, color-coded to match the beads in the abacus, provided an introduction to the ten nutrients studied. Children examined cells and carried out a number of other science activities. Many activities were also based on actual school lunch menus or on simulated school lunch situations.

The unit's effect was evaluated on the basis of scores on a pre- and post-test of nutrition knowledge—a modified version of Baker's test (1972)—and teacher and student comments. The raw scores were reported, but not the maximum possible for the test. All four groups exposed to the nutrition education unit showed a significant improvement in test scores ($p < .005$); the control group showed no such improvement ($p > .05$). No dietary or plate waste studies were attempted, since this was considered an exploratory study; and no immediate changes were thought likely from such a short unit.

Blakeway and Knickrehm (1978) designed a study to determine if a change in eating behavior, based on a nutrition education program, could be demonstrated through plate waste reduction in grades one, two, and three. The unit consisted of ten lessons, five of which emphasized tasting parties, and lasted an unreported time. The sample included about 5,000 students in 16 schools; 8 schools were randomly assigned to the control sample. Although nutrition education materials were made available to the control schools, they were given no special encouragement to use them. The experimental classes were given the materials plus the assistance of a nutrition educator (the developer of the unit), who took the major responsibility for teaching the unit.

In addition to classroom instruction on nutrition, the unit included tasting parties begun in the cafeteria and concluded in the classroom. Each of the parties was preceeded by a puppet show, developed and filmed by the nutrition educator, and an introductory talk by the cafeteria manager, thus fully integrating the school food service and classroom activities.

Plate waste was measured by grade before and after the nutrition education unit. Initially there was no difference in consumption between the two groups. The only change in the control was that grade one increased their consumption of sweet potatoes. In the experimental group, however, consumption of sweet potatoes in grades one and two rose significantly. Pinto beans were well accepted both before and after nutrition education; prunes were not. The researchers noted that although changes in acceptance for cottage cheese were statistically significant, the actual increase in amount was disappointing (from 1/4 to 1/3 ounce). The general trend of all the data pointed toward greater acceptance of previously unpopular commodity foods.

In a related study with kindergarten children, Blakeway (1977) found that emphasis on rutabaga in a unit tasting party led to its consumption by 59 percent to 69 percent of the children when served for the first time two weeks later. The study indicated that kindergarten, first, and second graders generally showed greater changes than third graders.

These studies seem to indicate that some behavioral changes can be brought about by nutrition education with young children when food experiences and instruction are integrated. However, the extent of the change must also be considered, since changes which are statistically significant may not always result in a sufficient practical improvement.

Cosper, Hayslip, and Foree (1977) reported a study conducted with two fifth grade classes of forty-five students, a majority of Mexican-American culture. The researchers developed eight thirty-minute nutrition education units on weight control. They then taught twenty-three students; the other twenty-two served as controls. The unit emphasized the importance of selecting proper foods for a balanced diet while reducing calories for weight control. Children took a forty-item nutrition knowledge test before and after the nutrition education unit; they also recorded their dietary intakes for a twenty-four-hour period.

Findings from the written pretest and posttest showed that the groups receiving nutrition instruction learned a greater number of nutrition concepts than did the control group ($p < .01$). The experimental group increased its mean score from 18.4 on the pretest to 21.8 on the posttest, out of a possible score of 40. Dietary intake records revealed that the diets of the experimental group did not improve after nutrition instruction. The mean dietary intakes were low for calories, calcium, iron, and thiamine both before and after instruction. The experimental group also had inadequate intake of vitamin A after the nutrition unit. Eighty-eight percent of the subjects had postdietary intakes that met less than 50 percent of the RDA for one or more nutrients.

This is another elementary school study in which there were

significant changes in nutrition knowledge, but not in dietary outcome. However, perhaps these students were not recording all that they were eating.

Shovic and Jennings (1979) designed a study with fourth graders to test whether a nutrition education program could increase nutrition knowledge, encourage vegetable acceptability, and reduce vegetable waste in school lunches. Approximately one hundred children in five classes participated in the five-week program. There was no mention of a control group nor of the frequency and duration of individual lessons. The ten-lesson program was especially devised to emphasize vegetables. The unit was activity-oriented and included vegetable tasting as well as instruction about the Basic Four, nutrients, the difference between nutritious and nonnutritious snacks, and a number of other topics.

The children scored significantly higher ($p < 0.01$) on the posttest compared with the pretest, reflected in a jump from 14.2 to 15.2 out of a possible score of 16. On the food acceptance questionnaire, there was a significant increase in acceptance of two vegetables out of the nine tested: cucumbers ($p < 0.05$) and cabbage ($p < 0.10$); these were among the three tasted by students during the program. There was no significant change in the amount of vegetable waste in school lunches before and after the program.

In this study, nutrition knowledge increased, and the opportunity to taste vegetables as part of the program was a positive influence on vegetable acceptance. Plate waste, however, was not influenced.

Tolin et al. (1979) compared two approaches to nutrition education with third graders, one based on food groups and the other on nutrients. A written test assessed nutrition knowledge, and plate waste in the school lunchroom was measured to determine any changes in eating behavior. Four classes of third grade students in two schools participated in the study. In each school one class of third graders served as the experimental group, and the other as the control group. The program consisted of ten thirty-minute lessons given on ten consecutive school days by the same instructor in both groups. One experimental group received instruction on the Basic Four, patterned after normal instruction in that school district. The other experimental class received instruction based on the five nutrients program designed by Nutrition Dynamics, Inc.

All the classes took a written nutrition knowledge test one week before the instruction period, immediately after the program, and six weeks later. The same test was used throughout, but with the order of the questions scrambled. Each test consisted of fifty four-option, multiple-choice questions: twenty-five to test material presented in the Basic Four instruction, and twenty-five to test material from the five nutrients instruction. The plate waste study was conducted for a three-day period, two weeks before and two weeks after the program.

On the five nutrients test section, the mean test scores on the post- and retention tests and the mean change in test scores from pre- to post-test were higher (p = 0.05) for the five nutrients experimental group than for either the other experimental group or the control groups.

On the Basic Four test portion, neither the nutrient approach nor the Basic Four approach improved students' scores. There was no difference between the posttest mean scores of experimental and control groups within each school or between schools.

The researchers summarized the results: "Students learned and retained more information on the five nutrients than on the four food groups, which indicated that they were capable of assimilating information on the five nutrients. Nutrition knowledge did not increase for students instructed on the four food groups" (1979). More accurately, the nutrient approach increased knowledge about nutrients from 30 percent correct on the pretest to 60 percent on the posttest and 48 percent on the retention test. The Basic Four approach did not increase knowledge about nutrients at all. The nutrient approach did not increase knowledge about the Basic Four on the posttest (58 percent correct on both pre- and post-tests) or on the retention test (61 percent). The Basic Four approach increased the knowledge about these food groups from 47 percent on the pretest to 49 percent on the posttest and 58 percent on the retention test—differences that were not statistically significant. Since the percent correct on all the tests seemed in the 50 percent to 60 percent range, it is unclear whether nutrition education was not very effective in either of the experimental groups, or whether the test instruments were inappropriate. Because of the variability of individual student participation in the school lunch program, it was impossible to determine whether instruction changed food consumption behavior as measured by plate waste.

Smith and Justice (1979) conducted a study to measure the influence of a student nutrition program, a parent nutrition program, and a combination of these two programs on the nutrition knowledge of third grade students, on their attitudes toward specific vegetables, and on their food practices at lunch. Twelve third grade classrooms in five elementary schools in an urban school system took part. Four classrooms were used to develop the evaluation instruments. Of the remaining eight classrooms, two were used for each of the following groups: control, parent education (PE), student education (SE), and parent education and student education (PE-SE).

The evaluation instruments were a written nutrition knowledge test consisting of twenty multiple-choice items, a hedonic scale with five different facial expressions used to measure the vegetable preferences of students, and a five-item lunch questionnaire measuring the eating habits of students. In two-week periods before and after the nutrition education programs, students took the nutrition knowledge test, the hedonic scale of vegetable preference, and the lunch questionnaire, the latter to be filled out each day after lunch for the two-week period.

The program for the SE group—four classes—consisted of eight forty-five-minute nutrition lessons taught for eight weeks, emphasizing vegetables. The program was activity-oriented: growing vegetables, playing nutrition games, solving puzzles, and feeling and tasting different vegetables of interest to the students. These activities were accompanied by discussions of the Basic Four, vegetables, and other aspects of nutrition. In the PE groups, students took home one letter a week for six weeks. In addition, these parents were invited to visit the lunch kitchen and to have lunch at school one day during the study.

On the nutrition knowledge test, no group showed any statistically significant increase in scores. The changes in mean rank scores on the vegetable preference scale were negative for the control group and positive, but not significant, for the experimental groups: for the SE group, $p > 0.05$ to $p < 0.1$; for the PE-SE group, $p > .01$ to $p < 0.2$. On the lunch questionnaire, there was a significant difference in participation in school lunch programs by the PE-SE group, and the consumption of vegetables at lunch by the PE group and the PE-SE group. Other significant changes varied by group. Parents of students in the PE group made favorable comments about the program.

Thus, unlike some similar studies, there was no significant improvement in cognitive knowledge. Trends toward more desirable nutritional behavior were suggested by the vegetable preference scores and some items of the lunch questionnaire, but they were not significant.

In a different kind of project, Talmage and Iverson (1979) used a case study approach to describe and identify factors and relationships in school food service that could change food attitudes and behaviors among elementary school children. Four urban public schools served as sites for structured observation and interviews. These case studies suggested that because food service plays a key role in one of the main eating events of the day—lunch—it can affect powerfully the students' food attitudes and habits. The researchers suggested that with collaborative efforts on the part of school food service personnel and teachers, the lunch program, like the educational program, may have a positive impact on students' food attitudes and behavior.

This study emphasizes that the presence of a school food service is in itself a nutrition education program, whether school personnel think of it that way or not. Without the cognitive mediation that is involved in classroom instruction, it can directly affect student attitudes and behavior. This factor must be considered in an evaluation of a nutrition education program.

Summary of Subjective and Objective Evaluations

Nutrition education today is undergoing change. Studies using subjective assessments report considerable enthusiasm among students, teachers, school food service workers, nutrition consultants, parents, and even school administrators.

Among the studies which used objective assessments to evaluate nutrition education, twelve out of thirteen relied on knowledge tests (see Table 1), with eleven showing gains in nutrition knowledge. Of those eleven, nine used statistics to analyze their results; the remaining two gave results in terms of percent increases from pre- to post-tests (ranging from 75 percent to 360 percent). Of the

Table 1
Evaluation Measures for Nutrition Education

Study	KNOWLEDGE Nutrition Information	Meal Selection	ATTITUDES Food Acceptance or Preferences	BEHAVIOR Food Record or Recall	Plate Waste	INVOLVEMENT WITH School Lunch (S) Community (C) Parents (P)
Lovett (1970)	+	+				C
Baker (1972)	+	+		0		
Boysen (1972)	+	+			0	
Bell (1973)	+		0		0	
Head (1974)	+	+ (5th grade)	+	0	+	S and C
	+	+ (7th grade)	0	+	0	
	+	0(10th grade)	0	0	0	
Jenkins (1975)	+					
Shoup (1975)	+			"Food feast" =?		
Wang (1975)	+	+	+			S
Myers (1977)	+	+				
Cosper (1977)	+	+		0		
Blakeway (1978)	+	+			+	S
Shovic (1979)	0	0	?		0	S
Smith (1979)	+		?		0/+	S and P
Tolin (1979)	+	+			?	S
Wodarski (1980)	+					

+ Item assessed; results positive.
0 Item assessed; results showed no change.
? Item assessed; results equivocal.

eleven studies which showed gains in knowledge, eight reported the maximum score possible. Four of the eight reported posttest scores in the range of 75 percent to 96 percent of the maximum possible score for four studies; the remaining four reported posttest scores in the range of 50 percent to 60 percent of the maximum possible. There is some question whether the low scores are due to ineffective nutrition education efforts (even with statistically significant gains in knowledge scores), or to tests that were inappropriate for the level of the learners or the task at hand (even though experts had screened and validated the tests).

Among the thirteen studies with objective assessments, four used measures of food acceptance or preference in addition to tests of nutrition knowledge. Of these four, two found no changes in preferences resulting from the nutrition education effort; the other two found only partial improvements in food acceptance.

Surprisingly, eleven of the thirteen studies used various behavioral measures to evaluate the nutrition education. Four of the six that measured plate waste found no changes, one found decreased waste of certain items, and another found decreased waste in one of the three grades tested. Four studies used dietary records or recalls; none was able to observe any change in the nutrient content of the foods selected following nutrition education, except for one study, which reported some changes in one grade out of three. A "food feast" in one study showed learning effects for two of the three experimental conditions. Another study employed a "lunch questionnaire," again with some improvements observed for a few items chosen for lunch. The sixth study measured height, weight, skinfold thickness, and arm and leg girth before and after the nutrition education program, but no changes in these parameters were attributable to the nutrition education unit.

All the studies using subjective assessments for evaluation were held in settings in which the school lunch program and classroom instruction were closely linked. Of the thirteen studies using objective assessment procedures, five used the school lunch to some extent—either by holding tasting parties using some of the vegetables served in the lunches or by planning and evaluating lunch menus.

Some of these programs illustrate the interrelationships among influences discussed in Chapter One. Of the thirteen, two programs were created in response to community surveys showing deficiencies of specific nutrients. One program was designed to address the problem of obesity that prevailed in a particular group. One study provided parent education; others sought parent evaluation but did not specifically offer parent education.

Even though there was overlapping between community and lunchroom involvement in some studies, seven of thirteen surveyed used neither the school lunch program nor community status information for nutrition education, although some of these seven did use plate waste studies to evaluate the effects of their efforts.

Conclusions Concerning Program Effectiveness

The finding that in eleven out of twelve studies nutrition knowledge gains occurred as a result of nutrition education, while only four out of eleven showed even small changes in food preference or behavioral measures is usually interpreted to mean that gains in nutrition knowledge are relatively easy to bring about, but desirable changes in nutrition attitudes and behavior are more difficult. While this is probably true, these studies alone do not provide adequate evidence; a number of factors must be considered in the interpretation of these results.

First, with one exception, these studies were all of relatively short duration. One was conducted over a period of five months, but neither the frequency nor duration of nutrition education events during this period was reported. The other studies were carried out over a period of two to ten weeks, with the majority in the three-to-six-week range. To expect a food behavior, which took years to shape and is reinforced daily, to change in a period of three to six weeks is unrealistic if not absurd.

Second, the timing of measurement of outcomes following an education unit is important since the benefits of nutrition education depend on time. For example, Green (1977) pointed out that an estimation of the effects can be influenced by the possibility of a delay of impact (the "sleeper effect"), a decay of impact (the "backsliding effect"), the start of an impact that would have occurred anyway ("borrowing from the future"), adjustment to trends in society, and a backlash from cessation of the programs.

In many of the studies reviewed, posttests were administered immediately after the unit, and then again six weeks later. Whether these are the best times to evaluate program effectiveness is not clear.

Third, some of the knowledge gains may be due to the "Hawthorne effect"—a change in behavior attributable to the special attention paid to subjects of an experiment and not to either the content or techniques of the program. Students may learn more, regardless of the teaching strategies, because the instruction and treatment of these students are not "business as usual."

Fourth, the measures themselves are problematic. Studies which described their nutrition knowledge tests indicated that the questions were of two general kinds: first, recall, comprehension, and application of information about nutrients, calories, and other aspects of the science of nutrition; second, ability to select or design a balanced meal. In the theoretical framework outlined earlier, we said that since one of the goals of nutrition education is to develop eating habits conducive to long-term health, the information must be useful in helping students make food choices consistent with this goal. The nutrition knowledge measures reported in the studies must be evaluated in terms of the usefulness of the information gained by students.

The actual questions asked on the tests were not reported, although examples were given in some cases. Children growing up with today's food supply need to worry less about deficiencies of major nutrients and more about deficiencies of trace elements and fiber, as well as excesses of calories, salt, sugar, and fat. Therefore, reported gains in knowledge about the major nutrients, deficiency symptoms, and food sources may not be meaningful even though they may be statistically significant. That is, food consumption learned as "one 2-oz. candy bar has 225 calories" is not nearly as useful as "one 2-ounce candy bar contains about as much sugar as three pounds of apples." Again, a student's increased ability to select balanced meals from items presented or to design balanced meals must also be interpreted in terms of the need to make food choices conducive to long-term health.

While the original purpose of the twenty-five-year-old Basic Four food guide was to ensure that people obtained sufficient amounts of protein, minerals, and vitamins in their diet, there are some failings; it does not distinguish well between foods in each group that are high in calories or fat and those that are low, nor does it distinguish between whole foods containing their full complement of trace nutrients and those containing only a fortified few. For example, the guide does not distinguish between a meal consisting of fish, broccoli, skimmed milk, and whole wheat bread, and a meal composed of hamburger, potato chips, a milk shake, and a white bread bun. The examples in the reviewed articles reflect this lack of distinction.

Furthermore, we were astounded to find that although the numbers of servings suggested for each of the Basic Four were not the same, test materials consistently asked students to choose *one item from each group* to balance a meal. This only leads to the implicit, if not explicit, message that half of one's food should come from animal sources (meat and dairy products). Such a pattern of eating can result in a diet excessively high in animal fat and protein, while low in fiber and in the trace nutrients found in plant foods. Although some have argued that the number of servings and the serving sizes stipulated by the Basic Four are a guide to good eating, others have noted that in practice many of the menus based on this guide are deficient in some of the essential nutrients (King et al. 1978).

Lastly, two kinds of behavioral measures were reported in the articles: food records and plate waste in the school lunch program. Both are problematic in evaluating nutrition education efforts.

The twenty-four-hour recall and record have problems too numerous to describe here, yet one troublesome issue is of particular importance. An individual's analysis of foods and snacks consumed in terms of the traditional nutrients (calories and the eight major nutrients) or in terms of the Basic Four does not tell us about the amounts of sugar, trace nutrients, fiber, saturated fat, and added salt in the diet.

Since self-reported behaviors are often inaccurate and nutrition-related behaviors typically are beyond the surveillance of school personnel, many nutrition education studies now use plate waste as a direct measure of food behavior. Plate waste studies tell us only that those particular foods, prepared in those particular ways, were or were not eaten on the days of measurement. They tell us nothing about changes in children's food habits in either desirable or undesirable directions. For example, children could be avoiding the corn-and-peas mixture in the school lunch, but eating enormous quantities of spinach salad, or no vegetables at all at home; there is no way for the nutrition educator or researcher to know which is the case. In those instances where a nutrition education unit emphasizes certain food items and provides opportunities for children to taste those foods, then plate waste measurement of those items is a valid measure of the effects of the unit. Nutrition educators must avoid an overemphasis on plate waste, which can turn nutrition education in the school into "school lunch menu item education." Therefore, we must be careful not to use evaluation instruments that are rigorously defined and quantitative, but which, unfortunately, yield results that are inappropriate or of no real significance in terms of the broader goal of developing desirable eating habits.

Implications for Nutrition Education with Children in Grades Kindergarten Through Six

The studies reviewed here provide little insight in how to achieve the goals of desirable nutrition knowledge, attitudes, and behavior; how to measure the results of nutrition education; or how to understand the relationships between these goals. Children need nutrition knowledge, both as part of a liberal education and for nutritional literacy in the face of an increasingly complex food supply. Using a variety of successful techniques, most of the studies reviewed here reported gains in nutrition knowledge. However, the articles were unclear as to how much of that knowledge was of an abstract, nutrition science/Basic Four variety and how much dealt with such issues as trace nutrients, additives, saturated fats, "junk food," and other realities of the U.S. marketplace. While appropriate knowledge does not in itself lead to appropriate behavior, it is certainly important for informed decision making.

Appropriate attitudes toward wholesome foods are also important to cultivate, although the studies showed we know little about how to cultivate such attitudes, nor do we know their precise relationship to behavior. While it is traditional to assume that knowledge influences attitude, which in turn influences behavior, rarely can we depend on this being true (Swanson 1972). Some researchers have found that in many instances "it is more likely that changing a behavior will change an attitude than that changing an attitude will change a behavior" (Evans and Hall 1978). We eat what we like, as has often been pointed out, but we also like what we eat. As an old commercial used to say, "Try it! You'll like it!"

In addition, all the attitude tests used in the studies reviewed here measured only stated food likes and dislikes or food acceptance (Birch 1979, Byer and Morris 1974). However, food likes or preferences represent only the affective dimension of attitudes, not the cognitive and behavioral dimensions (Zimbardo, Ebbeson, and Maslich 1979). Although the relationships among knowledge, attitudes, and behavior are complex, the cognitive and behavioral dimensions of attitudes are more predictive of actual behavior than is the affective dimension (McCullough 1980). For example, a person may report "liking" (affective dimension) ice cream, but "believe" (cognitive) that it is fattening, and thus rarely eat it (behavior). The behavioral component, representing behavioral intentions toward food (for example, intentions to purchase or to use), has been studied extensively by market researchers; it may also prove useful for assessments with children in the formal setting. Thus, the field of nutrition education urgently needs to devise imaginative, valid, and reliable measures of attitudes toward the complex issues of food and nutrition.

Desirable food behaviors are complex, embedded in many other aspects of a child's life. Classroom teaching alone will probably not bring about changes in behavior, nor will twenty-four-hour recall and plate waste data adequately measure them. Nutrition education may well need to explore strategies derived from other disciplines to bring about behavior change. Social learning theory (Bandura 1977), with its emphasis on vicarious learning through observation of model behavior, could probably be used with great profit in the classroom, in the lunchroom, and in the home to bring about desirable behaviors. Also, nutrition educators may need to explore evaluation procedures that go beyond those rooted in a social science whose paradigm is derived from the natural sciences. "Turning words into numbers, trends into prediction equations, and the behavior of people into probability tables or standardized regression coefficients" (Patton 1975) frequently fails to help us understand whether our nutrition education efforts have been effective in ways meaningful to the participants.

Consequently, nutrition educators must investigate the use of anthropological field techniques, such as participant observation, in-depth interviewing, detailed description, and qualitative field notes (Wilson 1979). One of the studies reviewed here used structured observations and field notes to investigate the influence of school food service on children's food choices (Talmage and Iverson 1979). Another reported some classroom techniques which could be useful to nutrition educators in the school (Sindell 1969).

CURRICULA AND PROGRAMS*

An enormous number of curricula and programs have been instituted by federal, state, and local educational agencies and by universities and food industry organizations. We have selected a few from each of the following categories: (1) state curricula, (2) comprehensive curricula designed by a variety of groups for nationwide use, and (3) innovative programs and curricula, perhaps originally designed for local use but now publicized or available nationwide as potential models for others.

As with the studies reported in the previous section, we evaluate these nutrition education curriculum guides and programs on the basis of whether they will develop childhood food consumption behavior conducive to long-term health; whether the teaching process will bring about not only gains in knowledge, but also the development of desirable attitudes and food behavior; and whether classroom learning is integrated with the lunchroom experience and with community resources. We also examine the readability and production quality of the materials, as well as the nature and usefulness of the information for teachers.

In general, current nutrition education curricula and programs in the schools are sequential to account for the cognitive, personal, and social development of children. In the early grades the objectives are to assist children in identifying and classifying foods and including a variety of foods in their diet. In the intermediate grades the emphasis is on nutrients, their functions in the body, and the psychosocial factors that influence nutritional behavior. In the

---

*Addresses for selected curricula and programs discussed in this section are listed in Appendix 2.

upper grades the focus is on applied nutrition topics of interest to adolescents, such as weight control and world food problems.

Researchers employ a variety of learning activities, such as discussions, cassettes, films, cooking, food tasting, and field trips, to accomplish the stated objectives. Evaluation procedures consist mostly of knowledge posttests at the end of lesson units. The more recent curricula emphasize application of knowledge and sometimes include attitudinal measures.

State Curricula

Most states now have, or are in the process of developing, comprehensive curriculum guides for statewide use. We selected a few that seemed representative of the full set of curriculum guides available for classroom use.

New York. The New York state curriculum was developed by the University of the State of New York and the New York State Education Department, Bureau of State Health Education and Services. Published in 1979, with minimum revision from an earlier edition, it is one component of the "Physical Dimension of Health Strand" of the State Health Education Program.

The teacher's manual for the elementary grades includes a section containing background information and two sections on learner objectives, concepts to be taught, learner activities, and evaluation procedures—one section for grades kindergarten through three and one for grades four through six.

The background information for teachers is extensive, consisting of about one hundred pages of information on the following topics: the evolution of food; eating behavior; nutrition science; effects of food on growth, development, and health; achieving and maintaining the best weight; teenagers' diets; nutritional needs in pregnancy; food ecology; nutritional problems in the United States; and global nutrition. Teacher information is also included throughout the text of the curriculum, paralleling the learner activities. Appendices give sources of nutrition education materials, describe common misconceptions about food and nutrition, and list the U.S. Dietary Goals.

The aims of the program are "to promote healthful nutrition

practices and to assist each person to overcome those personal or environmental factors that tend to interfere with the attainment of optimal nutrition." Emphasis is placed on the fact that "as the variety of foods available to us continues to increase, the ability to make intelligent choices among foods is of the utmost importance and becomes increasingly difficult." Fifteen goals are suggested emphasizing foods (as opposed to nutrients), the relationship between classroom activities and the school food service, and parent involvement.

The kindergarten through grade three section lists thirty-five concepts and understandings, as well as sixteen learner objectives for the four grades. Thirty-one "evaluative devices" are provided, which are intended to measure the comprehension acquired by students during their nutrition experiences in the primary grades. These devices must be used throughout the grades both to provide progress information and to ensure that all the competencies are achieved by the end of the third grade. The concepts and understandings to be taught are contained in three major topics (food development, food uses, and influences upon eating patterns) and four or five subtopics within each topic.

The grades four through six section lists twenty-five concepts and understandings and nineteen learner objectives implemented through about one hundred learner activities offered sequentially through the three grades. Forty-one "evaluative devices" are given for use in the three grades to measure whether learner comprehension has been achieved by the end of the intermediate grades.

The concepts and understandings are contained in five major topics: foods and civilizations, food selection and societies, how the body uses food, energy foods, and foods and growth. Background is provided not only on nutrition science but also on topics that are relevant to today's diet-related problems, such as obesity and heart disease. In addition to information on individual nutrients, food information is provided, and emphasis is placed on the importance of choosing foods that are minimally processed and low in fat. The Basic Four are deliberately ordered as the milk group, the grain group, the fruits and vegetables group, and the meat group in order to emphasize their relative importance. "Dietary Goals" are discussed as well as "junk foods," advertising, factors affecting overweight, teenage pregnancy, food assistance programs, ecological considerations, and other realities of the food system. The contextual material provided for teachers is useful for teaching children to make food choices that promote long-term health.

The topics and activities are food-based; nutrients are not emphasized until the upper elementary grades, where they are discussed in the context of food. As noted in the curriculum materials, "the more realistic the learning experience, the more likely that meaningful concepts will be developed . . . concepts upon which nutrition attitudes are established." The learner activities are numerous and are based on the child's real world. Classifying foods into the Basic Four is not an emphasized activity. In addition to the traditional stress on whole foods and science-type activities, others on snacks, school lunch, "junk foods," and advertising, are included.

The curriculum has some major weaknesses. The learner activities are generally good, but because the activities were derived with only minor revisions from an edition published ten years earlier, they fail to reflect changed perceptions about the nutrition education needs of children, needs so admirably discussed in the background information for teachers. Nor are the use of the school lunch program as a learning laboratory and parent involvement as prominent as the goals of the program suggest. The production quality of the materials is poor. Since no student worksheets are provided, teachers have to devise their own. The teachers' information, though highly relevant, is not very readable; only the highly motivated teacher could be expected to wade through the material. Thus, the curriculum places on the teacher a major responsibility to update the activities in light of the information in the manual and to design suitable worksheets. These factors undermine the usefulness of the curriculum guide in its present form.

Michigan. "Minimal Performance Objectives for Health Education for Michigan" was published by the Michigan State Department of Education in 1974. *Food—What's in It for You?*, a teacher reference guide for the nutrition strand, was developed by the Michigan Dietetic and Public Health Association in collaboration with the Department of Education, and was published in 1976.

The curriculum for the elementary grades consists of performance objectives and learner activities for two levels: Level I consists of grades one through three and Level II of grades four through six.

The overall concept for Level I is "We eat food to live." Five performance objectives are implemented through five subconcepts and thirty-six suggested experiences and activities. The overall concept for Level II is "We choose foods composed of different substances." Four performance objectives are launched through the teaching of four subconcepts, using about fifty suggested experiences and activities.

The background information for teachers consists of a twenty-page appendix containing information on the individual nutrients —their sources and functions—and on the Basic Four. Additional information, provided throughout the text, parallels the learner activities. The information for grades one through three consists of an elaboration of the Basic Four, and for grades four through six a discussion of the economic, psychological, and belief system effects on food choices, and of nutrients and their sources in the foods of various cultures. Resources, such as films, posters, and books, are included, along with the student activities.

Specific evaluation procedures are not given, but desired behavioral outcomes are listed. The teacher monitors these behaviors in the lunchroom or in parent-teacher conferences.

The suggested activities are typical of many other curriculum guides. The children play games, carry out experiments with foods, and learn about the Basic Four in the early grades; in the later grades they learn about their food habits, selection of a well-balanced diet, and appreciation of ethnic foods.

There are several other features to the Michigan curriculum. The school lunch and parent-teacher conferences are used in a few of the activities, thus integrating classroom learning slightly into other learning environments. No handouts for students are included, so teachers have to devise their own. The content of the nutrition education is far removed from the real experiences of the child. Like other materials developed before publication of the U.S. Dietary Goals, the Michigan curriculum does not provide the child with the kind of information useful for making food choices and developing eating habits conducive to long-term health in the context of today's food supply and nutrition problems.

West Virginia. The Child Nutrition Division of the West Virginia Department of Education is currently developing a curriculum for preschool and kindergarten through sixth grade. This comprehensive, sequential curriculum is based on the concepts proposed during the White House Conference on Food and Nutrition. The six major concepts are stated as "major generalizations," each of which is further elaborated into "specific generalizations" appropriate for children at different ages.

The major generalizations are: (1) "Nutrition involves the food people eat and the way the body uses it"; (2) "Food is made up of nutrients needed for growth and health"; (3) "All persons, throughout life, have a need for the same nutrients in varying amounts"; (4) "Food use by individuals and families is influenced not only by physiological needs, but also by cultural, social, economic, and psychological factors"; (5) "The way food is processed, stored, and prepared affects the amount of nutrients in it, its safety, appearance, and taste"; and (6) "Faulty or inadequate nutrition [malnutrition] is detrimental to health." Each of these generalizations is plugged into concepts geared to three levels: A, for ages five through seven; B, for ages eight and nine; and C, for ages ten and eleven.

At each level, these generalizations are implemented through the development of accompanying "essential competencies," as shown by appropriate "learner outcomes." That is, all the major generalizations are taught at Level A for grades one and two, repeated at a higher level of comprehension, B, in grades three and four, and taught again at a still higher level, C, in grades five and six. Numerous activities are suggested for each generalization to bring about the desired competencies. Evaluation procedures are given for each set of activities.

In the early grades the activities consist of identifying, classifying, and choosing balanced meals by means of games, food tasting, and role playing. In the higher grades activities include analyzing school lunch menus, role playing, digestion, individual nutrient needs, snacks, and influences on food use. Activities for grades five and six focus on the meaning of RDAs, the notion of "nutrient teamwork," food costs, food contamination, food additives, and nutrition labeling.

In general, the curriculum guide provides some information on foods and nutrition that takes into account the real world marketplace in which students must learn to make choices; teaches about practices which, if followed, are conducive to health; utilizes the school lunch experience; and provides for some contact with the home to reinforce classroom learning. The suggested evaluation measures test the ability to apply nutrition knowledge to contemporary situations and, indirectly, assess attitudes in some instances.

In general, this curriculum guide examines the concerns of nutrition educators today. Its major weakness is that discussions of these concerns are tacked on to an old framework—the White House Conference concepts and the Basic Four—whose content and implicit messages do not reinforce these concerns.

California. California is also designing a state nutrition education curriculum to replace previous ones. In the meantime the California State Department of Education has established "Minimum Proficiency Levels for Nutrition Education in California Schools," which support the nutrition concepts found in the "Health Instruction Framework for California Public Schools," adopted by the State Board of Education in 1977. These proficiency levels are intended as a foundation for nutrition instruction, curriculum development, and evaluation.

The curriculum consists of five topics (each with three to six subtopics), with minimum performance standards established for each, and graded according to the developmental levels of students in preschool through grade twelve. The topics are (1) food choices, (2) factors influencing food choices, (3) food-related careers, (4) consumer competencies, and (5) food handling.

In the lower grades children are expected to identify and classify foods, identify influences on food choices, understand the purposes of television ads, learn ways to prepare and handle foods, and identify people who work in food-related careers. In the upper elementary grades children identify the major nutrients, their food sources, and their functions in the body; how home and/or social eating environments influence food selection; ways of decreasing food waste at lunch; methods of handling foods in a sanitary manner to prevent illness and to maximize nutrient retention; and factors that affect the yield and quality of crops.

Developed by LEAs in California, these minimum proficiency levels have formed the basis of a number of curricula; two are described here for illustrative purposes.

The Rowland Unified School District developed a comprehensive, six-volume, sequential curriculum entitled *Energy Through Nutritive Basics.* Designed for students in preschool through grade six, the concepts are based on the student proficiency levels described above, and the materials were field tested. Each manual contains, in addition to a list of the proficiencies, suggested learning activities, multidisciplinary extensions, student materials, and sample lesson plans. Nutrition content information for teachers is provided throughout the manual. Teachers, food service employees, and parents are also provided with in-service nutrition information.

In the early grades the emphasis is on experiencing foods. Foods are discussed in terms of their plant parts, animal origins, and the traditional Basic Four. In the upper grades digestion and the roles and food sources of nutrients are introduced.

The strengths of the curriculum are numerous. The foods and activities are related closely to the real life experiences of the child. The implicit messages, more so than the explicit ones, take into consideration current diet-related nutrition problems. For example, the number of servings needed from each food group is emphasized repeatedly, so that children will not choose only one from each group. The order of the Basic Four is varied, avoiding implicit messages of relative importance. The activities and content also imply new ways of eating. For example, children discuss whole grains and legumes, grow sprouts, and make sprouted wheat muffins. The school lunch program is involved in activities to reduce food waste.

The curriculum's weaknesses arise from lost opportunities to reinforce some of these messages. For example, in the fifth grade unit on calories and energy, the importance of proper weight maintenance is not emphasized, yet this idea is first mentioned in the preschool/kindergarten unit. In addition, the fifth grade unit on changes in food habits could be improved by a discussion of the possible health consequences of current American eating patterns.

The production quality of the materials is good. The manuals do not have the slickness of commercially produced materials, but that means the materials are affordable by teachers and schools ($15 per volume). The student materials are suitable for reproduction and use by teachers.

The San Jose Unified School District also developed a comprehensive, sequential nutrition education program for preschool through grade six. Entitled *Please Pass the Nutrition,* the six-volume curriculum presents concepts that are based on the student proficiency levels established by the California State Department of Education and materials that have been field tested. The concepts are presented in four teaching units: "Nutrition Smart, Food Wise," "Type 'A' Everyday," "Kids as Consumers," and "Plants in the Making." According to the curriculum guides, "the major goal of the program is to develop a team approach to teaching and improving food habits of school children." Classroom experiences are designed for integration with school food service programs.

Each unit contains dozens of activities which meet the student performance objectives. Each activity is accompanied by a lesson objective and a list of required materials; teacher information and/or teaching considerations augment some of the lesson plans. In addition, instructional aids, such as sample handouts, miniposters, or worksheets, are attached to each lesson for easy use and for cost savings.

In the early grades, as with other curricula, children are provided with opportunities to taste and to classify foods, mainly using the Basic Four. The later grades are provided information on digestion, nutrients, food labeling, and a host of other topics. Food advertising, "junk food," and other real world issues are included, although not to any great extent.

As with other recently developed curricula, the program is strongly activity-oriented. Many of the activities involve the school lunch program, so that the integration between classroom and cafeteria is quite extensive. Teachers can use the numerous handouts directly, and the curriculum guides are affordable (about $15 per volume). The materials seem a little difficult for the age group intended. For example, nutrients are introduced early in the program. Discussions of today's diet-related health problems are not detailed enough to be maximally useful for developing eating habits conducive to long-term health.

Comprehensive Curricula Designed for Nationwide Use

Several curricula have been developed in the past five years by universities and food industry trade associations for nationwide use.

FOOD . . . Your Choice. Over the years, the National Dairy Council (NDC) has produced a number of materials and program packages that are widely used in American schools. In 1975 NDC began developing a comprehensive and sequential curriculum for elementary and secondary schools. After conducting a needs assessment and analyzing the existing nutrition curricula, a committee of consultants was formed to guide the process of curriculum design and field testing. The result of this study is *FOOD . . . Your Choice,* described as a "Nutrition Learning System." The grades one through six segment became generally available in 1977 and is now used in some 150,000 classrooms with about 4.5 million children. The segment planned for use with high school students is in the design stage.

The materials point out that "Nutrition education should prepare students to make intelligent food choices and to establish healthful dietary habits." The curriculum assists students in clarifying the effects that social, psychological, and physiological factors have on food choices and emphasizes the notion of individual choice. The key ideas of the curriculum are based on the concepts proposed during the White House Conference (noted in the description of the West Virginia curriculum).

The key ideas derived from these concepts and used for organizing the curriculum are: "Nutrition: Effect of Food on Energy, Growth, and Health"; "Nutrients: Their Relationship to Health"; "Food Handling: Its Effects on Health and Food Quality"; "The Life Cycle: Its Effect on Nutritional Needs of People"; "Social/Psychological Needs: The Influence on Food Choices"; "Food Technology: Its Impact on the Food Supply"; and "Nutrition and Society: An Interdependence."

These key nutrition concepts are introduced at the primary level and further developed in the later grades. The three sequential programs in the curriculum are designed to take into account the intellectual, personal, and social development of the students at different ages. The curriculum is multicultural and can be used in all subject areas in the school curriculum. Level One introduces five- to seven-year-olds to basic nutrition concepts: Why do I eat? What do I eat? Where does my food come from? When and how much do I eat? Level Two extends these concepts for eight- and nine-year-olds by considering the power of food, food comparison and clarification, food life-styles, and food consequences. Level

Three is designed to assist ten- to twelve-year-olds in decision making by studying nutrients in food and factors that influence eating patterns and food choices.

In the early years children are given the opportunity to taste and appreciate food. In the middle years the emphasis is on classification of foods into the Basic Four food groups. In the upper elementary grades the subject of nutrients is emphasized, as well as such related issues as food labeling. Value clarification (beliefs about foods) is carried out with students at several points during the program, under the stated assumption that "Values—one's beliefs and attitudes—determine behavior."

At each level there are two to four units of instruction containing numerous learning activities. In each unit the objectives are stated in behavioral terms. The teaching strategy is, by design, activity-centered so that students have the opportunity to acquire information through the manipulation of materials. Each unit also has a knowledge posttest for students and an evaluation checklist for teachers.

The nutrition education program was evaluated in 1977-1978, using four schools in each of five school districts representing five U.S. geographic regions and different socioeconomic levels (Talmage 1978). One hundred and four teachers and thirty-five hundred students participated in the study. The complex evaluation study provided built-in control groups without depriving any students of the opportunity to receive nutrition instruction. A comparison of students' pretest and posttest scores on a "Nutrition Achievement Test" revealed statistically significant gains in nutrition knowledge. Nutrition attitudes and food choice behavior were obtained from the less rigorous evaluative measure of teachers' subjective impressions of student attitudes and behavior. All teachers reported indications of improvements in these areas. For example, teachers reported that students brought more nutritious snacks to school and were more likely to discuss the nutritional value of their meals. Teachers evaluated the program favorably and found they could easily incorporate the material into other subject areas with little disruption. A high percentage of teachers reorder the materials each year.

The program has several strengths. It provides a sequential, systematic, and comprehensive approach to nutrition. Its emphasis on activities generates interest, motivation, and the opportunity to develop inquiry skills. The units can be easily integrated into the other subjects in the school curriculum, and the nutrition information is scientifically accurate. The materials are of high production quality; student materials contain spirit masters and other materials which can be directly used by the teacher. Although very little nutrition information is provided in the teacher's manual, teachers are trained to use the materials. The program is provided to teachers at nominal cost, and the student materials can be renewed yearly. Take-home materials, consisting of letters to parents and nutrition information leaflets, are provided in an effort to link instruction in the classroom with food practices in the home.

The program's major weakness is that it does not provide enough of the kinds of information that would enable children to make food choices conducive to long-term health. The Basic Four is emphasized, and distinctions are not made between those foods within each group that are high in fat and added sugar or salt. Furthermore, since the curriculum planners made the policy decision that there are no such things as "junk foods" and that all foods are good when eaten in the proper amounts, healthy snacks are emphasized; however, the materials also include the less healthy snacks commonly consumed by children. The net effect is that the curriculum is not very useful in guiding students to make appropriate food choices (the stated goal of the program) in the real world marketplace.

Big Ideas in Nutrition Education. This nutrition education curriculum, originally developed by the Dairy Council of California in the early 1970s, now forms the basis of the nutrition education program of Dairy Council, Inc. (DCI), headquartered in San Antonio, Texas. DCI's network of seventeen offices serves the seven-state region in the South and Southwest. During the 1978–79 school year, nearly one million school children completed the *Big Ideas* program (Zuber and Moerchen 1979). Eventually the program will be available throughout the United States and Canada (Fisk 1979).

Based almost entirely on teaching the Basic Four, the program has been described as "the leanest, most specific set of objectives to help students learn this one ability: how to assess daily food intake" (Shortridge 1976). Others call it "a basic, no frills education unit that teaches students the nutrition skills they will need to lead a healthy life" (Zuber and Moerchen 1979).

The *Big Ideas* curriculum consists of the following units:

1. "Little Ideas" teaches preschool children to accept a wide variety of foods. It includes a set of 105 colored food pictures and activities for preparing peanut butter, pudding, butter, stew, and ice cream.

2. "Balanced Meals" is the primary unit (for second graders), which teaches students how to nutritionally balance a meal by including "at least one food from each of the four food groups." A leaflet is provided for parents, and students bring workbooks home at the end of the unit.

3. "Daily Food Choices" is an intermediate unit for the fifth grade. In addition to reviewing the food classification skills learned in the earlier unit, students learn the number of servings needed and serving sizes.

4. "Teen-age Nutrition Program" teaches students to select nutritious foods when eating away from home by checking how many additional servings, if any, are needed to meet minimum recommended amounts for each of the four food groups.

The educational philosophy of the program is that it should *not* be integrated with other subjects in the curriculum "since it can cause confusion or ineffective learning in the classroom" (Fisk 1979).

Big Ideas units come complete with student workbooks, pre- and post-tests, classroom visual materials, and detailed guides. Teachers are also provided training in use of the materials. The production quality of the materials is good, and they can be used directly by school teachers.

The program has been widely field tested and evaluated (Lovett, Barker, and Marcus 1970; Fisk 1979; Zuber and Moerchen 1979; Cooper and Philp 1974; Niedermeyer and Moncrief 1975; Dickey 1976). It is a competency-based program, so that while many of these studies report results in terms of improvements in scores, others do so in terms of the percent of students who achieve 80 percent mastery. Reteaching, through remedial exercises, can increase the level of mastery to 95 percent of students. In those studies reporting scores, the figures ranged from about 40 to 50 percent on the pretest to 80 to 90 percent on the posttests (Zuber and Moerchen 1979, Fisk 1976). In terms of the mastery level achieved, at least 80 percent of the learners master the basic food

ation and selection skills, at the 80 percent level (Zuber and en 1979, Fisk 1976). In one study breakfast consumption ere gathered with third graders, but little change was found (Lovett, Barker, and Marcus 1970). Food consumption data gathered with teenagers showed "a marked increase in the number of students who included recommended minimum servings in their daily food selections" (Zuber and Moerchen 1979).

The major weakness of the program is that it focuses narrowly on teaching the Basic Four. Materials do not distinguish foods within each group that are high in calories, fat, or added sugar from those that are low. Also, in the primary unit, where students are given practice in selecting balanced meals, children are repeatedly asked to choose *one* food from each group. These two shortcomings in the material are likely to result in food choices that are high in animal foods and low in plant foods, and that may contain more calories than necessary within food categories.

Nutrition Education in a Changing World. Pennsylvania State University, under the sponsorship of the Nutrition Foundation and with the support of the Heinz Endowment, is in the process of developing a comprehensive nutrition curriculum for preschool through grade twelve. The overall goal of the curriculum is "to produce high school graduates who, after exposure to nutrition education for 12 or more years, can think, feel and perform in a nutritionally literate manner in making decisions for themselves and others" (*Nutrition Education in a Changing World* 1978).

In generating the curriculum's concepts and skills, a team of experts formulated "40 project learner objectives" to embody the skill, knowledge, and attitude areas considered crucial to good nutrition decision making for the target high school graduate. These learner objectives were submitted to 1,000 members of the Society for Nutrition Education to evaluate and rank. The following four objectives were given the highest ranking:

1. Analyze one's own nutrition and food patterns, identify problems, if any, and initiate action to correct those problems.
2. Describe the relationship between nutrition and health.
3. Be able to explain why the inclusion of a variety of foods in the diet is desirable.

4. Critically evaluate food and nutrition claims on a logical and nutritionally informed basis (Barnette and Branca 1978).

These and the other learner objectives were incorporated into a framework designed to answer the following questions: Why do we need nutrition? What nutrients do we need and how much? How do we get our nutrients? How do our nutritional needs change? How do we study nutrition? (Sherman, Lewis, and Guthrie 1978)

The teacher's manual explains the rationale behind the unit sequencing:

The units are organized into a spiral curriculum format, but with dimension shifts. Pre-schoolers accumulate first-hand experience to broaden their perspective of what variety of things may be considered as foods. Primary students have shown that they can indeed understand and apply nutrient concepts, and are expected to learn the foods containing a few nutrients. Intermediate students should be able to perform analyses of nutrients from composition tables and guide their own progress in precise ways. (*Nutrition Education in a Changing World* 1978)

In the primary units the concepts and activities are designed to help children become "informed nutrition consumers," "eager and educated eaters," and "wise and critical selectors" of foods. The following precepts are enunciated: "A good diet can include all kinds of food, depending upon personal preference and budget. Natural, fabricated or convenience foods, as well as the more traditional ones, can have their place if one knows how to choose a good diet." "Each time we eat, we must decide what to eat. A wise selection of foods at meals and in between can add up to a total diet that meets individual needs, as well as personal preferences." Activities revolve around food variety, nutritious eating, and "Where shall we eat out?"

The intermediate units emphasize the body (digestion, and so forth) and nutrients. Activities are designed to assist students in identifying the food sources of various nutrients and in making personal choices recognizing that "nutrition is a matter of deciding degree rather than making all-or-none selections from extreme views."

The goals of each unit are stated in behavioral terms, and each lesson includes specific learner objectives. Teachers are expected to adapt the numerous activities to suit the needs of a given class. The student worksheets and quizzes that are provided can be easily copied for classroom use. In addition to making a cognitive "post-assessment" for each lesson, teachers are encouraged to note informally any behavioral changes exhibited or reported. Background information is provided in the curriculum materials.

An evaluation of the *Changing World* curriculum and of three different types of teacher preparation on the nutrition knowledge of students in kindergarten through grade six was carried out with just under 3,000 students in 29 schools in Pennsylvania (Shannon et al. 1980). Teachers (124 in all) were divided into three groups: those who used only the information in curriculum guides, those who attended a three-hour in-service session in addition, and those who took a three-credit nutrition course in addition to attending the in-service session and using the curricular information.

In all grades the mean knowledge gains of children taught nutrition via the curriculum was higher than gains of children in comparable control groups (using an analysis of variance). Teacher preparation had a significant effect only in grades four and six. In the fourth grade, students of teachers who had taken the course tended to perform best, but in the sixth grade, students of teachers who had attended only the in-service session did best. Most of the 754 parents who completed a survey questionnaire reported that their children were talking at home about what foods do for the body and/or the Basic Four food groups. Almost all favored the nutrition education program.

As in the other more recently developed curricula, *Nutrition Education in a Changing World* is comprehensive, sequential, and based on expertise derived from a number of disciplines. The activities are adequately described for a teacher to follow. Worksheets are provided and the production quality is good, the information scientifically accurate, and the approach balanced. Activities involving the school food service are also included.

Similar to the other new programs, the curriculum content does take into consideration some of the realities of today's eating environment, such as snacking and television ads; these issues are explored in some detail in the junior and senior high school units. In the elementary school units, however, the emphasis is on the major nutrients and their utilization and roles in the body. It is unfortunate that other relevant nutrients, such as saturated fat, sugar, salt, fiber, and trace elements, are not included, nor is much mention made of the problem of overweight. The fault, again, lies with the Basic Four food group system. The curriculum's viewpoint is that there are no such things as "junk foods," only "junk diets," and that providing information on the major nutrients is sufficient for children to be able to choose from among all foods nutritious, "non-junk" diets. This weakness in the curriculum content is ameliorated somewhat by the emphasis on the importance of eating a variety of foods. Its moderate stance also appeals to many nutrition educators as appropriate in light of uncertainties about interpreting the scientific data.

Nutrient Density–Nutrition Education Curriculum. This comprehensive curriculum for students in kindergarten through grade six is based on the concept of nutrient density and the Index of Nutritional Quality (INQ), which is a means of measuring a food's nutritive value based on a comparison of its nutrients to energy or calorie content (Sorenson and Hansen 1975). The program, according to the introduction, "does not tell students what they can or cannot eat. Such rules too often impose unacceptable or unreasonable dietary restrictions. Instead, students are encouraged to 'mix and match' foods to meet their nutrient needs within calorie requirements while satisfying their own individual taste preferences. This approach to dietary selection allows for the use of non-traditional food combinations and encourages the use of ethnic foods." Nutrient principles are discussed through the use of food profile cards, listing the content of eight nutrients and total calories for each of several hundred foods. Students learn to use transparent overlays to perform nutrient addition, thereby evaluating foods on the basis of their nutrient composition and selecting foods which are nutritionally complementary by balancing the strengths and weaknesses of individual foods.

The program is divided into three units: Unit I for kindergarten through grade one, Unit II for grades two and three, and Unit III for grades four through six. The teacher's manual for each unit contains explanations of the program and specific instructions for teaching the unit, concepts and behavioral objectives to be taught, and detailed plans for some thirty lessons at each unit level. Students in grades two through six receive skill books, or workbooks, file cards for 128 foods. In addition, the teacher's *Index of Nutritional Quality Food Profiles Master-* ʼe nutrient density profiles of over 600 foods.

̱ʌ̣ᴄ concepts and behavioral objectives were established ̱ʲ ᴛwenty nutrition educators who reviewed the literature and the White House Conference concepts. A concept emphasized throughout is: "The food profile card indicates a food's nutritional value." The following concepts are included in Unit I: "Understanding nutrition begins with recognition of and interest in a variety of foods"; and "Grouping nutritionally related foods is an important first step in understanding the concept of a balanced meal." Unit II concepts are: "Nutrients play important roles in maintaining health"; "A variety of foods in the diet is necessary for good health"; "Food undergoes changes in the digestive system"; and "Food labels give useful information." Unit III, in addition to reinforcing knowledge about nutrients, emphasizes food labeling and INQ nutrient addition, application of nutrition knowledge in day-to-day situations, and designing meals that are nutritionally adequate and that take into account sociocultural factors.

The program was evaluated in 9 public elementary schools in Utah and Idaho with 806 students in 27 classrooms (Brown, Wyse, and Hansen 1979). The teachers attended a one-day intensive workshop in solving problems that illustrated program concepts. The units were used as an integrated part of the elementary school program. Pre- and post-tests were conducted in addition to classroom evaluations. At all grade levels, 80 percent or more of the students performed at the 80 percent accuracy level or above on their ability to use the food profile cards to find a food's nutritional value, and on their ability to carry out nutrient addition and nutrient complementation (grades two through six). In addition to increased knowledge about the nutritional quality of foods, students showed greater acceptance of high-nutrient density foods and less acceptance of low-density foods on a food preference test. Posttest scores on an attitudinal survey of students in grades four through six were also slightly improved over pretest scores.

The developers of the curriculum were quite aware of both the strengths and weaknesses of the nutrient density approach. Some nutrition educators have suspected that teaching about the Basic Four food groups through several grades has in the past turned off a large proportion of students. The major strength of this program is that, by enabling students to assess individual foods, it retains their interest and is probably also a more effective means of teaching nutrition, given contemporary eating patterns and the increased ability of students to cope with scientific knowledge. The school lunch is utilized as a teaching tool, with students both analyzing and planning school menus. Finally, the nutrient density approach takes into account those thousands of food products on the supermarket shelves which today do not fit into the food group system.

The greatest weakness of the curriculum results from the use of only nine selected nutrients. Students could come to believe that only nine nutrients are required for optimal health. More seriously, the use of these particular nutrients is based on the notion that they are "indicator" nutrients. Eight to ten standard nutrients used to be enough to judge the nutritional value of a food. If a diet of whole foods had adequate amounts of these indicator nutrients, it could be assumed that the diet was adequate in the forty or so others as well. But if a significant proportion of the daily intake of the indicator nutrients is supplied by highly fortified, processed, or fabricated foods, the indicator system is no longer of value. It cannot distinguish, for example, between broccoli and sawdust fortified with the same amounts of six or eight of the major nutrients found in broccoli. The presence of other nutrients—especially trace nutrients, which are so easily lost in processing—cannot be assumed from such nutrient calculations. However, if a nutrient density approach is well used, it should bring out these issues.

One other factor needs further consideration. The developers assume that children today are capable of greater scientific sophistication than their parents, and that once they have mastered the skills of nutrient addition and complementation using transparent overlays, they have learned about nutrients. That assumption requires further exploration, in light of one study indicating that most children interviewed outside the formal school setting did not spontaneously mention nutrients in relation to the fate of foods inside the body; among the few who did, even fewer demonstrated an understanding of the words (Contento 1980).

Comprehensive School Food Service–Related Nutrition Education Curriculum. In 1976 the Food and Nutrition Service of the USDA contracted with Applied Management Associates to develop a food service–related nutrition education program for students in kindergarten through grade twelve and to evaluate the impact of all components of this program on students' knowledge, attitudes, and opinions about food; food selection practices at school and away from school; participation in the school lunch program; and acceptance of the foods served.

A comprehensive review of the literature and interviews with food service personnel led to selection of the White House Conference concepts for the curriculum, with special emphasis on two: "Food is made up of nutrients, each of which has a specific function in the body," and "All foods provide a variety of nutrients and no one food can provide all the nutrients necessary for health." To these was added the following: "The Type A lunch provides approximately 1/3 of a student's daily requirements for most nutrients."

These concepts are divided into three units: Basic Nutrition, Consumer Education, and Health. Each unit is composed of five lessons. The precise content is geared to the behavioral and social interests of the age groups. The Basic Nutrition Unit teaches about the nutrients, their functions, food sources, and body requirements for nutrients. It serves as a foundation for the other units. The Consumer Unit in the lower grades concentrates on where foods come from, how they are processed, and how they get to the consumer. In the Health Unit the topic areas in the lower grades include food safety and sanitation, and in the middle grades, nutrition and dental health. All the units employ the discovery approach to learning. Learning strategies include role playing, scientific and laboratory experiments, analytical problem solving, games, and puzzles.

In all, the curriculum consists of sixteen books containing not only classroom-oriented activities but also those related to the school food service program. In addition to a manual for teachers, which is traditional with all curricula, a manual for school food service managers is provided as a companion package to the teachers' units. For each unit, three to six supplementary activities, complete with spirit masters, teaching aids, and background information, utilize the resources of the manager and/or the cafeteria/kitchen.

The curriculum was field tested before implementation. It was evaluated in 5 school districts in 5 states, involving 30 schools, 6,268 students, 183 teachers, and 30 school food service managers.

The thirty schools were divided into treatment and control groups. During the test period of about five months, the effects of the curriculum on the National School Lunch Program were assessed by five evaluation instruments: knowledge tests, food preference and acceptability tests, school lunch participation rates, and plate waste records.

According to the summative evaluation of the program, significant statistical gains in nutrition knowledge took place among students for all three units at all grades; no similar gains were noted for the control students. There was no overall significant positive or negative effect on students' behavior toward food at school or away from school. In grades kindergarten through three, in particular, there were positive changes in certain individual attitudinal scale items, such as choosing healthy snacks, the importance of exercise, and advertising. The plate waste observations demonstrated overall, but not statistically significant, increased consumption of school lunch by experimental students, with statistically significant increases in consumption of meat, milk, bread, and "other" foods (for example, dessert and potato chips) for most grade levels. Teachers evaluated the program favorably, and food service managers reported that use of the activities helped improve their relationships with teachers and students.

Innovative Curricula and Programs

We now turn to five recent innovative programs, originally designed for local use, but whose contents have become widely publicized as models for others, or whose curricular materials are available. Evaluations of these programs are included, where possible.

The Learning for Life Program.   This program was a response to the concern of parents, teachers, administrators, and others in the Newton, Massachusetts, area about the relationship of eating patterns, exercise, and various personal stress-coping behaviors to health. Since modifications of such behaviors in later life can be quite difficult, members of the Newton community requested that the schools provide more and better health education so that young children could be assisted in acquiring the knowledge and attitudes that might help them form beneficial lifetime eating and exercise patterns. The program was designed to "encourage desirable life-time practices in the areas of nutrition and physical fitness through a study of the interrelationships between physiology, nutrition, and exercise" (Newton Public Schools 1979). ESEA Title IV-C funded the program, and the Kellogg Foundation funded its evaluation. This nutrition and fitness program consists of two curriculum components: *The Dufus Stories* is for second (or third) graders, and *From the Inside Out* is to be used in upper elementary classrooms.

The Dufus Stories, an 88-page book of stories conveying nutrition and fitness concepts, is designed to be read to second grade children. It is accompanied by a teacher's guide and resource manual—a 218-page volume containing background information; about 100 student activities; and 52 worksheets, puzzles, and noncompetitive fitness games, coordinated with the chapters in the Dufus Stories. Word cards and posters are also included. The format of having teachers read stories to students was chosen because the rudimentary reading skills of most second graders make it difficult to use the printed word to convey any but the simplest ideas. The activities were chosen to introduce children to the complexity of decision making and the many factors—peer pressure, advertising, family background, personal preferences—that can influence behavior. The activities involve the supermarket, the home, the streets, and the classroom. Parents are involved through a series of informative handouts sent home periodically during the eight to ten weeks of the curriculum.

From the Inside Out is a 220-page volume of nutrition and fitness information and concepts presented in readable fashion for upper elementary children. It is accompanied by a 218-page teacher's guide and resource manual containing background information, dozens of student activities, and resource information; and a 197-page student workbook containing games, puzzles, and worksheets. The curriculum is planned as a sixteen-week unit, taught in one classroom period daily and two physical education sessions weekly. However, the program can be extended to a year or condensed to suit individual classroom needs. Parent information sheets are provided and several activities are designed around parent-child interaction.

The second grade program (*The Dufus Stories*) was evaluated to assess whether second graders increased their knowledge about nutrition, body function, and exercise; whether they developed positive attitudes toward proper nutrition and physical fitness, and improved their physical fitness; and whether parents of participating students increased their awareness of good nutrition and physical fitness.

Seven experimental and seven control schools were randomly selected for the evaluation. Within each school, one second grade class was selected by the school. Tests of nutrition knowledge and attitudes were developed and administered before and after the program, and again six months later. Despite uncertainty at the outset whether the program would produce measurable differences in behavior between experimental and control groups over the short time span of the experiment, a simple running test was administered to assess the fitness objectives of the program, and a snack survey was used to evaluate the food habit objectives of the program. A parent questionnaire, a teacher questionnaire, and student interviews were also administered.

Significant gains in knowledge and in positive attitudes were found for the experimental group, both immediately after the conclusion of the program and six months later. The snack survey, which was logistically complex, revealed no significant differences in the composition of snacks eaten by experimental and control group students. Likewise, there were no significant differences in the posttest running scores between the two groups. Students, parents, and teachers were highly enthusiastic about the program.

This is not a comprehensive kindergarten through sixth grade program, but it appears to be one of the best. The information and activities are very "real," based as they are on realities of the world in which children have to make their life-style choices. The curriculum also is built around information and activities that are useful in developing the knowledge, attitudes, and habits conducive to long-term health in the context of today's nutrition- and exercise-related health problems. This is done not only explicitly, but implicitly as well. For example, the Basic Four approach is used, but the importance of relative serving numbers is emphasized by activities calling for children to balance meals not by filling in four squares, but by filling in boxes arranged thus:
The vegetable/fruit and grain groups are always pictured or de-

scribed first, followed by the milk group and the meat/bean/eggs group to emphasize their relative importance. Within each of the four groups, foods are further subdivided into those that can be eaten "any time," those that should be eaten "sometimes," and those that should be eaten only "now and then." Information is given in terms that have real meaning for youngsters, such as "one 12-ounce can of soft drink contains 8 tablespoons of sugar." It is a food-based curriculum. Snacks, food labels, the history of foods, the parts of plants and animals various foods come from, food comsumption data, and food composition data are presented in interesting fashion. Nutrients are discussed but not emphasized.

The activities reinforce the implicit and explicit messages of the nutrition information. For example, children grow vegetable gardens and make whole wheat bread and cheese instead of high-sugar, high-fat, baked items. The integration of nutrition and physical fitness presents a more holistic approach to the issues of healthy life-styles.

The only weakness of the curriculum is that although the reading level was judged to be appropriate for the students in the Newton school district, it may prove too difficult for students in some other locations. The school food service is not included specifically in the activities, because so many children in the Newton schools bring their own lunch.

Lady Bugs and Lettuce Leaves. This is a gardening and environmental education curriculum component of PROJECT OUTSIDE/INSIDE, which was developed by the Somerville, Massachusetts, Public Schools with funding from the Massachusetts ESEA Title IV-C program, the Somerville School District, and CETA. The project is a curriculum development and community information program in health, nutrition, and gardening.

A curriculum for fifth and sixth graders, *Lady Bugs and Lettuce Leaves* is aimed at developing an awareness of the interrelationships within the environment and an understanding of plant growth through the planting of a garden; nutrition is one of the components. The curriculum consists of a 45-page text, including concepts and instruction for hands-on activities, and a 103-page teacher's manual; it draws on the resources of workshops and garden specialists. The nutrition unit emphasizes the vegetable garden as a source of plant foods containing the various nutrients, and

familiarizes children with the plant parts that serve as
curriculum could form an excellent complement to class.
trition education and the school lunch experience.

The Food Education Project. A food curriculum for the primary grades was developed by the University of Hawaii, under the
sponsorship of the Hawaii State Department of Education and with
funding from the Consumers Education Program of ESEA (PL
93–380). The concepts and activities for the curriculum were a
response to in-depth interviews with 144 parents of first and third
graders in Honolulu. While the parents wanted their children to
learn from various food experiences, they were primarily concerned with the safety of an activity and its educational value.
Parents also felt that children should develop independence as
they progressed from simple food activities to those of increasing
difficulty.

The goal of the food curriculum is to teach children about food
and its place in the human experience, and it focuses on the often-
neglected aspects of food. At the primary level, the curriculum is
an interdisciplinary program consisting of four units: The Lunch
Table at School; the School Garden; To Market, To Market; and
Seashore Foods. The teacher's manual describes the program thus:

> The table is where foods are served. In the unit on *The Lunch
> Table at School* children study the food prepared and served
> in the school cafeteria. Gardens are where foods are grown
> and *The School Garden* unit involves sprouting seeds and
> growing plants of nutritional value. The market is where
> families in Hawaii acquire most of their food. In *To Market,
> To Market* children write shopping lists and purchase the
> items listed at a local market. The beach is where some nutri-
> tious food from plants can be gathered by young children. Sea
> and seashore vegetables are collected and studied as part of
> the *Seashore Foods* unit. (Food Education Project 1978)

The food curriculum is firmly rooted in child development concepts. The activities are planned to progress from the table at home
to the neighborhood market and ultimately to the seashore. The
curriculum helps children develop food vocabularies, increase
their skills in working with food, and become familiar with their
food supply. These considerations are particularly important in a
society where many children grow up thinking that "grains" are

manufactured in factories and that "cooking" consists of dropping plastic bags of frozen vegetables into boiling water. This program also firmly involves parents in the process of curriculum planning and in the child's ongoing activities with food, so that the classroom and home complement each other. The school lunch experience is also fully integrated with classroom food activities.

This project is exemplary in that it reminds nutritionists that people eat food, not nutrients, and that there are many ways of thinking about food. Indeed, the designers of the program argue that nutrition education should teach children how to think about food—that is, how to "use symbols appropriate for communicating about food" and to analyze "those food systems which impact on their own lives." In an era when foods are changing rapidly, this process should lay "the foundation for a lifetime of decision making" (Maretzki 1979).

The School Health Curriculum Project (The Berkeley Project). Over the past 20 years, this prototype health education program has developed from a project in one classroom (sixth grade) in one school district to a fairly comprehensive program (grades two through seven) which has been implemented in about 300 school districts in some 30 states and in 2 international locations. It contains a nutrition component in the fourth grade (Evans and Middleton 1979).

The goal of the program is to help students understand the functioning of their own bodies, what affects health, and how to make personal decisions about their own health and life-styles. The program is designed to use existing materials and to involve family and community members and agencies in addition to the school. It is strongly activity-based, with activities related to other subjects and to many aspects of the student's immediate world. The emotional arena is stressed, as well as the social and physical, and students are encouraged to develop self-concepts. A one- to two-week training workshop for teachers and health educators is the main vehicle for successful implementation of the program.

The nutrition component for the fourth grade explores the effects of behavior on health.

With an emphasis on nutrition and the digestive system, students learn about energy and chemical interactions within the body. By designing charts, mobiles, and displays depicting the various nutrients and their jobs, students learn the importance of food choices on their total health. As a follow-up activity, parents are invited to a breakfast planned by students which emphasizes essential nutrients. Consumer issues, environmental pollution, immunization, and personal medical care are also explored in this unit. (Evans and Middleton 1979)

The grades five through seven units have been validated by the U.S. Office of Education and evaluated by a number of researchers, who found positive changes in attitudes and behaviors, although most of the measurements were in the area of smoking (Olsen, Redican, and Krus 1980). The grades kindergarten through four units, containing the nutrition component, have not been validated. Nevertheless, the program is interesting and nutrition educators should be aware of its existence.

Nutritional Wild Edibles. This ESEA Title IV-C program in Calhoun County, West Virginia, is designed to introduce students, parents, and teachers to "an almost lost art known to the early pioneers." According to its materials, "the project pays unhesitating homage to the late Euell Gibbons who popularized wild culinary arts." The program is based on the notion that urbanization and the resulting pollution are rapidly reducing the American wilderness, including its wild edible plants. Identification and cultivation of genuine natural foods are skills that are considered too valuable to be lost. Thus the program seeks to involve both parents and students in locating, identifying, preparing, and tasting the wild edibles of West Virginia. From these activities, students learn about nutrition, as well as the need to protect the environment.

Although we have not seen any validation data, the program is included here as an example of the rather unusual kind of learning experience which more nutrition educators should be creating.

Creative Food Experiences for Children. Originally written for the Community Coordinated Child Care Council and the Montgomery County Health Department, this volume is included because it has become the unofficial curriculum guide in many schools throughout the country.

The guide teaches elementary children about food and nutrition through numerous activities in which children prepare, taste, and understand food. Children work systematically with vegetables, fruits, milk, protein foods, and grains and cereals. The activities emphasize whole grains; alternate protein foods; bread and yogurt preparation; sprout growing; and concern about highly processed food products and those containing large amounts of fat, sugar, or salt. The information is comprehensive, and the activities take into account the food supply and children's experiences in today's society. The guide is useful for introducing children to traditional whole foods and to alternate ways of eating—ways that may enhance long-term health.

SUMMARY AND CONCLUSIONS

The curricula and programs reviewed here were chosen because they either were widely publicized or seemed typical of other curricula. They were evaluated on the basis of whether the content would be useful to youngsters seeking to develop life-styles conducive to long-term health and whether the teaching process integrated learning in the classroom with other locations in which children eat. These studies were also evaluated on the basis of improvement, both in nutrition knowledge and in desirable attitudes toward food and sound eating behavior.

Of the eleven comprehensive curricula and programs reviewed, seven stated desired outcomes in terms of competencies or proficiencies, and three in terms of learning outcomes or some comparable, more broadly defined behavior. One curriculum used a discovery approach and did not list specified behavioral outcomes. Eight involved the school food service to some degree, four of them extensively. One was designed specifically as an integrated nutrition and physical fitness program. Ten of the eleven were designed to be integrated into other subject areas but one should instead be taught by itself. Almost all (nine out of eleven) were field tested before implementation. The more recently developed curriculum materials are a dramatic improvement over those available in 1976, when Cooper and Go conducted an exhaustive review of curriculum guides (Cooper and Go 1976).

Because measuring behavioral change is so difficult, most field testing measured student knowledge gains and the extent of favorable responses among parents and teachers. Field evaluation data were available for six of the eleven curricula; of these six, all found that students gained in nutrition knowledge (compared with a matched control group). Three field evaluations systematically and formally measured attitude change and found that positive changes occurred as a result of the programs. However, most of the test items either measured food preferences or directly elicited opinions. Four of the six attempted to measure behavioral change in some formal manner but were generally unable to detect any changes that were attributable to the program. However, we may not yet have devised appropriate measures of nutritional behavior. Plate waste measurement in the school lunchroom and snack surveys are rarely as sophisticated as the instruments used for measuring knowledge and attitudes. Furthermore, a longitudinal study may be the only fair test of the impact of six years of nutrition education on elementary school children.

In terms of nutrition education content, three of the eleven curricula selected concepts from the 1969 White House Conference. One program was based almost entirely on teaching the Basic Four. The remaining programs derived their conceptual frameworks either from surveys of professional nutrition educators or from gleaning the nutrition education literature. These concepts were implemented mostly through the traditional four food group/nutrients approach, although the curricular approaches spanned the spectrum from largely nutrient to largely foods.

Throughout our review, we evaluated the usefulness of the nutrition information presented in the curricula. We emphasized this aspect because, although most educators would agree that nutrition education should prepare young people "to make intelligent food choices and to establish healthful dietary practices," what is meant by "intelligent food choices" or "healthful dietary practices" is often unclear. Such statements must be interpreted and judged in terms of the ultimate goal of nutrition education: the production of a healthy citizenry in the context of today's nutrition-related health problems and the current food supply.

As nutrition educators, we must constantly remind ourselves that definitions of usefulness change over the years because of the changing contexts in which "healthful" food choices have to be made. Earlier in this century, people were urged to eat more calories and protein; later, they were urged to add to their diets foods high in vitamins and minerals. Out of a concern for the widespread deficiencies of the major nutrients came the impetus to fortify processed and fabricated foods. The curricula of past decades reflect this concern: the Basic Four, nutrients, and the White House Conference concepts. We must not abandon our concern with nutrient deficiencies, but we must also be concerned about the excessive amounts of fat, sugar, and salt, and inadequate amounts of fiber and possibly trace nutrients in the diet of most Americans. Nutrition curricula should reflect these concerns, and we must also recognize that they too are bound to change over time.

The curricula varied from four which made little or no mention of these concerns to two which were based on them; most lay somewhere in between these two extremes. Seven curricula discussed "junk foods" and other realities of today's marketplace; four did not. In some instances the discussion appeared to be tacked on to a conceptual framework that did not account for these issues. In only three, surprisingly, these issues were integrated into the curriculum through such activities as emphasizing whole grains and legumes. Nor was eating the right amount of food to maintain weight emphasized. In general, the innovative, locally developed programs were more comprehensive in their coverage of these issues.

In terms of educational approach, all curricula were intended to assist children in making wise choices and developing good eating behavior. Three stressed decision making as the goal of nutrition education and value clarification. The assumption behind this approach is the Rogerian notion that "humans are basically good, social and forward-looking, who, given freedom" and given adequate information, "will in the end adopt these behaviors which are positive and rational" (Kolbe 1979). Or the assumption is that education should provide extensive information on the issues but should never interfere with an individual's freedom of choice.

Other curricula more explicitly encouraged the consumption of certain foods and discouraged the consumption of others. These programs take a Skinnerian approach, perceiving individuals as less than truly free to adopt those behaviors which would be most healthy in light of the numerous forces in society urging the public, often in quite scientific and sophisticated ways, to behave otherwise (Kolbe 1979). Therefore, these programs tend to draw more on persuasion-communication techniques to influence attitudes and behaviors. The majority of the curricula and programs used a mix of both these philosophical approaches, failing to notice that they make fundamentally different assumptions about the learner and the learning process.

For two reasons nutrition education cannot consist solely of the value-free, objective process of providing scientifically accurate information about foods and nutrition so that children can choose foods freely on the basis of a cost-benefit analysis of each food. First, no usable curriculum for children can provide all the needed information about every food product for truly informed decision making. Since some facts are included and others are not, the curriculum is not value-free. For example, by providing information on the major nutrients in a food but omitting information on its fat or added sugar and salt content, and the risk-benefit ratio of each of its naturally present or added carcinogens, the curriculum has already limited the decision-making ability of the students. Second, if nutrition education programs and curricula continue to be evaluated according to their effects on the behavior of children, it must be assumed that we believe some behaviors are more desirable than others. Nutrition education cannot avoid specifying what these are and why they are desirable.

Does this mean then that nutrition education should concern itself with propagandizing rather than educating (Moore 1978)? We do not think so. True, we must provide children with the knowledge and decision-making skills that will enable them to choose between this food and that. But we must also teach them how to think in ways that will enable them to understand the health effects, energy costs, ecological consequences, and moral implications of their food choices; how to analyze the impact of the food system on society as a whole; and how to act self-reliantly in providing nourishing meals for themselves and others. Those who seek to educate the young must design creative curricula and learning strategies so that such teaching can be accomplished.

BIBLIOGRAPHY

Abraham, S., and Nordsieck, M. 1960. Relationship of Excess Weight in Children and Adults. *U.S. Public Health Service Public Health Reports* 75:263.

Baker, M.J. 1972. Influence of Nutrition Education on Fourth and Fifth Graders. *J. Nutr. Educ.* 4:55.

Bandura, A. 1977. *Social Learning Theory.* Englewood Cliffs, N.J.: Prentice-Hall.

Barnette, J.J., and Branca, M. 1978. Learner Objectives for a Nutrition Education Curriculum. Part Two—Factor Analysis. *J. Nutr. Educ.* 10:65.

Bell, C.G., and Lamb, M.W. 1973. Nutrition Education and Dietary Behavior of Fifth Graders. *J. Nutr. Educ.* 5:196.

Birch, L.L. 1979. Preschool Children's Food Preferences and Consumption Patterns. *J. Nutr. Educ.* 11:189.

Blakeway, S.F. 1977. Journey through Foodland: One District's Nutrition Project. *School Food Service J.* (July/August): 110.

Blakeway, S.F., and Knickrehm, M.E. 1978. Nutrition Education in the Little Rock School Lunch Program. *J. Amer. Dietet. Assoc.* 72:389.

Bosley, B. 1947. A Practical Approach to Nutrition Education for Children. *J. Amer. Dietet. Assoc.* 23:304.

Boysen, S.C., and Ahrens, R.A. 1972. Nutrition Instruction and Lunch Surveys with Second Graders. *J. Nutr. Educ.* 4:172.

Brown G.; Wyse, B.W.; and Hansen, R.G. 1979. A Nutrient Density–Nutrition Education Program for Elementary Schools. *J. Nutr. Educ.* 11:31.

Byer, N.R., and Morris, P.M. 1974. Food Attitudes and Snacking Patterns of Young Children. *J. Nutr. Educ.* 6:131.

Contento, I. 1980. Children's Thinking About Food and Eating—A Piagetian-Based Study. Paper presented at the Workshop on Nutrition Education Research, Cornell University, Ithaca, N.Y., April 28–30.

Cook, C.B.; Eiler, D.A.; and Kaminaka, E.C. 1974. How Much Nutrition Education in Grades K–6? *J. Nutr. Educ.* 6:99.

Cooper, B., and Philp, M. 1974. Evaluation of Nutrition Education in Everyday Teaching Environment. *J. Nutr. Educ.* 6:99.

Cooper, D.A., and Go, C.E. 1976. Analysis of Nutrition Curriculum Guides at the K–12 Level. *J. Nutr. Educ.* 8:62.

Cosper, B.A.; Hayslip, D.E., and Foree, S.B. 1977. The Effect of Nutrition Education on Dietary Habits of Fifth-Graders. *J. of Sch. Health* (October): 475.

Creswell. 1913. Girls' Club Work in Georgia for 1912. *Georgia State College Agric. Bull.* 1, no. 6.

DeZeeuw, M.L. 1979. Discover Nutrition Education Through SACs. *School Food Service J.* (June/July): 96–106.

Dickey, R. 1976. Keeping Nutrition in Mind. *School Food Service J.* (July/August): 103.

Dobbins, F.W. 1971. Nutrition Education Through School Food Service. In *Proceedings of the National Nutrition Education Conference*, Misc. Publ. no. 1254. Washington, D.C.: U.S. Department of Agriculture, p. 56.

Eagles, J.A.; Pye, O.F.; and Taylor, C.M. 1979. *Mary Swartz Rose, 1874–1941, Pioneer in Nutrition*. New York: Teachers College Press.

Education Commission of the States. 1975. *The Status of Nutrition Education*. Denver: Education Commission of the States.

Evans, N.L., and Middleton, K.H. 1979. Two Programs Exemplify Nationwide Involvement in School Health Education. *Health Educ.* (November/December): 42.

Evans, R.I., and Hall, Y. 1978. Social-Psychologic Perspective in Motivating Changes in Eating Behavior. *J. Am. Dietet. Assoc.* 72:378.

Fisk, D. 1979. A Successful Program for Changing Children's Eating Habits. *Nutrition Today* (May/June): 6.

Food Education Project. 1978. Honolulu: State Department of Education.

Foster, T.A. et al. 1977. Anthropometric and Maturation Measurements of Children Ages 5 to 14, in a Biracial Community—The Bogalusa Heart Study. *Am. J. Clin. Nutr.* 30:582.

Frank, G.C.; Berenson, G.S.; and Webber, L.S. 1978. Dietary Studies and the Relationship of Diet to Cardiovascular Disease Risk Factor Variables in 10-Year-Old Children—The Bogalusa Heart Study. *Am. J. Clin. Nutr.* 31:328.

Garn, S.M. et al. 1975. Growth, Body Composition, and Development of Obese and Lean Children. In *Childhood Obesity,* vol. 3, ed M. Winick. New York: John Wiley & Sons.

George, J.C. 1971. A Nutrition Education Unit for a Sixth Grade. *J. Nutr. Educ.* 2:111.

Gonzales, N.W. 1969. Changing Dietary Patterns of North American Indians. In *Nutrition, Growth and Development of North American Indian Children,* eds. W.M. Moore, M.M. Silverber, and M.S. Read. DHEW Pub. no. (NIH) 72-26.

Green, L.W. 1977. Evaluation and Measurement: Some Dilemmas for Health Education. *Am. J. Pub. Health* 67:155.

Halfacre, M. 1977. Why Johnny Eats. *School Food Service J.* (October): 70.

Head, M.K. 1974. A Nutrition Education Program at Three Grade Levels. *J. Nutr. Educ.* 56.

Hegsted, M. 1979. Interview quoted in Nutrition and Health, by H.J. Anders. *Chem. and Eng. News* (March 26): 27.

Jenkins, S.; Stumo, M.; and Voichick, J. 1975. Evaluation of the Nutrition Film Series "Mulligan Stew." *J. Nutr. Educ.* 7:17.

Johnson, C.L., and Abraham, S. 1979. Hemoglobin and Selected Iron-Related Findings of Persons 1–74 Years of Age: United States, 1971–74. *Advancedata* (Newsletter of the U.S. Dept. of Health, Education, and Welfare) 46:1.

Johnson, M.J., and Butler, J.L. 1975. Where is Nutrition Education in U.S. Public Schools? *J. Nutr. Educ.* 7:20.

Kamhi, M.M. 1980. Making Diets Healthy at P.S. 166. *Nutrition Action* 7:3.

King, C. 1979. Take the Team Approach to Nutrition Education. *School Food Service J.* (October): 76.

King, J.C. et al. 1978. Evaluation and Modification of the Basic Four Food Guide. *J. Nutr. Educ.* 10:27.

Kolbe, L.J. 1979. Evaluating Effectiveness—The Problems of Behavioral Criteria. *Health Educ.* (January/February): 12.

Langworthy, C.F. 1913. Home Economics Work for Boys and Men. *J. Home Econ.* 5:239.

Legget, A.L. 1913. The Introduction of Home Economics in a South Carolina Rural School. *J. Home Econ.* 5:139.

Lovett R.; Barker, E.; and Marcus, B. 1970. The Effect of a Nutrition Education Program at the Second Grade Level. *J. Nutr. Educ.* 2:81.

Lucas, B. 1977. Nutrition and the Adolescent. In *Nutrition in Infancy and Childhood.* St. Louis: C.V. Mosby Co.

Maretzki, A.N. 1979. A Perspective on Nutrition Education and Training. *J. Nutr. Educ.* 11:176.

Martin, J. 1978. School Nutrition Programs in Perspective. *J. Amer. Dietet. Assoc.* 73:389.

Mayer, J., ed. 1969. Weight Control in Public School Children. *Postgraduate Medicine* (June): 267.

McCullough, J. 1980. Attitude Research in Consumer Behavior. Paper presented at the Symposium on Attitude Theory and Measurement in Food and Nutrition Research, Pennsylvania State University, June 15–17.

McKenzie, J.C., and Mumford, P. 1965. The Evaluation of Nutrition Education Programmes: A Review of the Present Situation. *World Rev. Nutr. and Dietetics* 5:21.

Meyers, L.D., and Jansen, G.R. 1977. A Nutrient Approach in the Fifth Grade. *J. Nutr. Educ.* 9:127.

Moore, J.L. 1978. Nutrition Education: Propagandizing vs. Merchandising. Speech presented at the Eleventh Annual Meeting of the Society for Nutrition Education July 17.

Mullins, A.G. 1958. The Prognosis in Juvenile Obesity. *Arch. Dis. Child.* 33:307.

National Nutrition Policy Study. 1974. Hearings Before the Select Committee of the U.S. Senate 93rd Congress, on Nutrition and Human Needs. Second session, Part 3—Nutrition and Special Groups, Part 4—Nutrition and Native Americans.

National Research Council. 1974. *Recommended Dietary Allowances.* 8th rev. ed. Washington, D.C.: National Academy of Sciences.

Newton Public Schools. 1979. *Evaluation of the Title IV-C Learning for Life Program.* Newton, Mass.: Newton Public Schools (July).

Niedermeyer, F.C., and Moncrief, M.H. 1975. Primary-Graders Study Nutrition. *Elem. School J.* (February): 305.

Nutrition Education in a Changing World. 1978. University Park, Penn.: The School Nutrition Curriculum Study of Pennsylvania State University.

Nutrition Education is as Easy as 1, 2, . . . 9. 1976. *School Foodservice J.* (July/August): 57.

Nutrition Today. 1972. Highlights from the Ten-State Nutrition Survey. *Nutrition Today* (July/August): 4.

Olsen, L.K.; Redican, K.J.; and Krus, P.H. 1980. The School Health Curriculum Project: A Review of Research Studies. *Health Educ.* (January/February): 16.

Patton, M.Q. 1975. Alternative Evaluation Research Paradigm. Grand Forks, North Dakota: North Dakota Study Group, Center for Teaching and Learning, University of North Dakota.

Picardi, S.M., and Pariser, E.R. 1975. Food and Nutrition Mini-course for 11th and 12th Grades. *J. Nutr. Educ.* 7:25.

Powers, M.A. 1978. Health and Nutrition Activity Under Title IV Part C of the Elementary and Secondary Education Act. Washington, D.C.: U.S. Office of Education, October 6.

Reese, W.J. 1980. After Bread, Education: Nutrition and Urban School Children, 1890–1920. *Teachers College Record* (May).

Rizek, R.L., and Jackson, E.M. 1980. Current Food Consumption Practices. Paper presented at the International Conference on Implementing the Dietary Guidelines: The Potential for Food Product Development, sponsored by the American Health Foundation, May 14.

Roberts, L. 1927. *Nutrition Work with Children.* Chicago: University of Chicago Press.

Robinson, C.H. 1976. Nutrition Education—What Comes Next? *J. Am. Dietet. Assoc.* 69:126.

Rose, M. S. 1932. *Teaching Nutrition to Boys and Girls.* New York: Macmillan.

Shannon, B. et al. 1980. A Nutrition Education Study, Grades 4–6: Curriculum and Teacher Preparation Effects. Unpublished manuscript. Pennsylvania State University.

Sherman, A.R.; Lewis, K.J.; and Guthrie, H.A. 1978. Learner Objectives for a Nutrition Education Curriculum. Part One—Identification and Priority Ranking. *J. Nutr. Educ.* 10:63.

Shortridge, R.C. 1976. Learner Success or Failure? *J. Nutr. Educ.* 8:18.

Shovic, A.M., and Jennings, G. 1979. Effects of Nutrition Education on Nutrition Knowledge, Vegetable Acceptability, and Plate Waste. *School Food Service Res. Rev.* 3:21.

Sindell, P.S. 1969. Anthropological Approaches to the Study of Education. *Rev. of Educ. Res.* 39:593.

Smith, H.M., and Justice, C.L. 1979. Effects of Nutrition Programs on Third Grade Students. *J. Nutr. Educ.* 11:92.

Sorenson, A.W., and Hansen, R.G. 1975. Index of Food Quality. *J. Nutr. Educ.* 7:53.

Strunkard, A. et al. 1972. Influence of Social Class on Obesity and Thinness in Children. *J. Am. Med. Assoc.* 221:529.

Swanson, J.C. 1972. Second Thoughts on Knowledge and Attitude Effects upon Behavior. *J. Sch. Health* 42:363.

Talmage, H., and Iverson, B.K. 1979. A Look at School Food Services in Influencing Food Choices: Cases and Instruments. *School Food Service Res. Rev.* 3:65.

Talmage, H. et al. 1978. *FOOD . . . Your Choice, Levels 1, 2, and 3.* Summative Evaluation. Technical Report 98. Office of Evaluation Research. Chicago: University of Illinois at Chicago Circle.

Tolin, D. et al. 1979. A Comparison of Two Approaches to Nutrition Education at the Third Grade Level. *School Food Service Res. Rev.* 3:24–28.

Ullrich, H.D. 1979. Towards a National Nutrition Education Policy. *J. Nutr. Educ.* 11:60.

U.S. Department of Health, Education, and Welfare. 1975. Preliminary Findings of the First Health and Nutrition Examination Survey, United States, 1971–72: Anthropometric and Clinical Findings. DHEW Pub. no. (HRA) 75–1229. Rockville, Maryland: National Center for Health Statistics, April.

———. 1972. Ten-State Nutrition Survey, 1968–1970. Atlanta: Center for Disease Control.

———. 1978 Total Serum Cholesterol Levels of Children 4–17 Years. DHEW Pub no. (PHS) 78–1655. Hyattsville, Maryland: National Center for Health Statistics.

U.S. Senate Select Committee on Nutrition and Human Needs. 1977. Dietary Goals for the United States. 2nd ed. USGPO no. 052-070-04376-8 (December).

Vegetables on Parade. 1979. *School Food Service J.* (October): 50.

Wang, M., and Dwyer, J.T. 1975. Reaching Chinese-American Children with Nutrition Education. *J. Nutr. Educ.* 7:145.

White House Conference on Food, Nutrition, and Health. 1970. Section Four, Panel 1: Nutrition Teaching in Elementary and High Schools. *J. Nutr. Educ.* 1:24.

Whitehead, F.E. 1957. Nutrition Education for Children in the United States Since 1900. Parts I and II. *J. Amer. Dietet. Assoc.* 33:880.

———. 1970. Nutrition Education Research Project: Report of Phase I. Washington, D.C.: Agency for International Development, Office of Nutrition, Technical Assistance Bureau.

Wilson, C.S. 1979. Food—Custom and Nurture: An Annotated Bibliography on Sociocultural and Biocultural Aspects of Nutrition. *J. Nutr. Educ.* Supp. 1.

Wodarski, L.A. et al. 1980. Teaching Nutrition by Teams-Games-Tournaments. *J. Nutr. Educ.* 12:61.

Zimbardo, P.G.; Ebbesen, E.B.; and Maslich, C. 1979.*Influencing Attitudes and Changing Behavior.* Reading, Mass.: Addison-Wesley.

Zuber, S., and Moerchen, B.D. 1979. Nutrition Education: It's a Winner! *School Foodservice J.* (August): 63.

Zumsteg, D. 1976. From Celery to Zucchini, It's All Part of Learning. *School Foodservice J.* (March): 53.

7

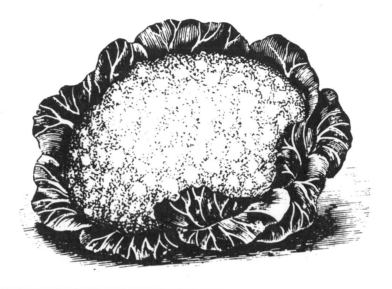

SECONDARY
SCHOOL
NUTRITION
EDUCATION

Martha L. Plass and Martha C. Mapes

INTRODUCTION

This review examines nutrition education in the secondary school setting and describes those intervention programs which have been subject to evaluation. Our examination also reveals effective nutrition education approaches and points to areas where further effort is needed both in programming and in research.

Many of the risks to adolescent health are inherent in modern American culture. Schools can and do play a significant part in influencing health-related behaviors; however, as stated in the Surgeon General's report, *Healthy People,* "The task of health promotion and disease prevention for adolescents is . . . multi-faceted, requiring the contributions of a wide range of health professionals and evaluators—and perhaps more importantly, the family and peer group" (Institute of Medicine 1979). With this qualification in mind, the Surgeon General's report suggests that organizations such as schools, where young people gather for reasons unrelated to health, have special promise for health and nutrition education.

To answer the basic question of how the school can play a role in producing nutritionally sound behavior, we first review the background data on adolescence which can serve as a basis for targeting programming. In the second part of the chapter we describe current programs designed to meet the needs of adolescents and offer recommendations for programming and research.

BACKGROUND DATA

The following three areas are especially important to consider in planning for nutrition and health education: (1) nutritional requirements and status, (2) biological implications of growth and maturation, and (3) psychological aspects of adolescence.

Nutritional Requirements and Status

Research on nutrient needs indicates that growth and maturation are influenced by environmental factors, and that nutrient and caloric requirements increase during the growth spurt. For example, age of menarche may be influenced by nutrition status (Valadian 1971). Dietary zinc deficiency has also been shown to retard growth and sexual maturation (McKigney and Munro 1976). Height and weight may be affected, but the adolescent human body seems to be capable of maintaining growth with wide variation in caloric intake (Valadian 1971, Hegsted 1976). Further complicating the problem of determining requirements, caloric and nutrient needs decline as the growth rate slows, usually by the age of thirteen in females and sixteen in males. Therefore, for many individuals, caloric needs start to decrease during adolescence.

A comprehensive bank of knowledge about actual nutrient needs during adolescence is missing in today's research. In fact, at the Airlie Conference in 1973 nutritional scientists stressed this problem (McKigney and Munro 1976). In summarizing the data on nutrient status, Hodges (1976) noted that "the most commonly neglected nutrients appear to be iron and vitamin A, although riboflavin, calcium, and pyrodoxine may also be in short supply." As Hegsted (1976) observed, "the best summary one can make about the calorie, fat, protein, and amino acid needs of adolescents is that there are so few factual data for this age group and that nearly everything we presumably know is obtained by extrapolation."

The most recent advances in knowledge regarding status have come from the Health and Nutrition Examination Survey (HANES) data indicating the extent to which nutrient needs are being met. Other recent data on adolescence have been gleaned from the Ten-State Nutrition Survey, the 1965 Household Consumption Survey, and the 1977–78 Nationwide Food Consumption Survey (NFCS).

The HANES study, conducted from 1971 to 1974, measured the nutritional status of a scientifically designed sample of the civilian, noninstitutionalized U.S. population. The only national assessment of its kind, the HANES study included a general medical examination by a physician for indicators of nutritional deficiency, skin examination by a dermatologist, dental examination by a dentist, body measurements, a dietary interview consisting of a food frequency questionnaire and a twenty-four-hour diet recall, a medical history, and numerous laboratory tests for biochemical analysis (U.S. Department of Health, Education, and Welfare 1976, 1979c). Although vast amounts of HANES data are still being analyzed, initial reports provide some information on the nutritional status of the U. S. adolescent population.

The Nationwide Food Consumption Survey, also using a national population sample, gathered information from households on food used, food intake of individual members, family composition, education and employment of the head of household, participation in food programs, and other factors which might affect food consumption (Hama 1979). The twenty-four-hour diet recall, in conjunction with a participant's record of food consumption for the next two days, was used to assess dietary intake.

Although other reliable studies of nutrition status have been conducted with smaller population samples (Huenemann et al. 1968; Hodges and Krehl 1965; Wharton, 1963; U.S. Department of Health, Education, and Welfare 1972), none has examined a sample that is statistically representative of all U.S. age, sex, ethnic, and income groups. Many of the findings from these studies using smaller samples reiterate the HANES and NFCS results.

These surveys must be interpreted, however, in light of the standards for nutritional adequacy that they use. These standards are set using the best available knowledge about adolescent nutrient requirements. Most surveys, including NFCS (Pao 1979), use RDAs as the basis for assessing dietary adequacy. HANES uses some of the RDAs and also has established other, similar standards (U.S. Department of Health, Education, and Welfare 1979 b). The RDAs are based on available date concerning nutrient requirements for the majority of the population; the lack of information on adolescent requirements has made establishment of RDAs for this age group difficult. The initial decision to divide adolescents into two age groups (ages eleven to fourteen and fifteen to eighteen) categorizes adolescents into junior and senior high age groups rather than into physical maturation groups (Mueller 1976). Many of the values in the RDAs for adolescents are derived from the "judgement factor" and extrapolations from infant and adult data (Hegsted 1976, Mueller 1976). Consequently, evaluations of adolescent dietary intake based on RDAs are difficult to assess for accuracy (Hegsted 1976, Leverton 1968). In addition, older surveys of dietary intake use older RDA values, which have since been changed because of new nutrition knowledge. Re-evaluations of past data demonstrate that adolescent populations thought to have had inadequate intakes have adequate intakes according to newer

RDAs. Other dietary surveys have used the Basic Four food groups to assess adequacy; this approach is problematic, since some foods can be classified in more than one food group, distorting the data (Leverton 1968). Finally, it must be recognized that most individuals within a population will be perfectly healthy despite intakes below the recommended levels.

Other problems with standards and methodology exist in any nutritional status survey. However, the data collected from HANES and NFCS still present the best information now available.

Calories. HANES found that *caloric intake* peaked in fifteen- to seventeen-year-old males and ten- to eleven-year-old females (U.S. Department of Health, Education, and Welfare 1979b). This age range corresponds to the adolescent growth spurt, when caloric requirements would be highest. The 1979 NFCS reported highest caloric intakes at fifteen to eighteen years in males and twelve to fourteen years in females (1979). These caloric intakes were lower than those found in the 1965 survey. Both HANES and NFCS reported caloric intake below the recommended level for adolescents, but NFCS found similar mean body weights in 1965 and 1978. HANES reported that caloric intakes below standard did not correspond to the distribution of lean and obese persons in the subgroups. These discrepancies may be due in part to reporting biases in the diet recall method or to differences in physical activity levels. Further analysis of HANES data will indicate whether reduced caloric intake is reflected in adolescent growth performance. Also not yet reported is the degree of obesity in the adolescent population.

In regard to the *sources and distribution of calories,* the NFCS preliminary analysis indicated that absolute protein intake was highest in fifteen- to eighteen-year-old males, but was down from 1965 in all age-sex groups (Pao 1979). Despite the reduction in average protein intake, the percentage of calories from protein had increased slightly since 1965. The largest mean intake of fat was also recorded in the fifteen- to eighteen-year-old male group. Both average fat intake and percentage of calories derived from fat were lower than in 1965, but were still above the level recommended (Pao 1979).

Overall carbohydrate consumption dropped between 1965 and

1978, but the proportion of calories was up. Again, the same adolescent male group had the highest mean intake. Unfortunately, the type of carbohydrate, simple or complex, is not mentioned.

So far, only mean intakes of protein are reported from HANES, and these met the standards for all adolescents except white females in the low-income group. The proportion of those who did not meet the dietary standards ranged from 23 to 26 percent of males and from 41 to 58 percent of females (U.S. Department of Health, Education, and Welfare 1979b). Future reports from HANES will analyze carbohydrate and fat intakes in adolescents.

Vitamins. NFCS reported that mean intakes of *vitamin A* for all age-sex groups were sufficient to meet recommended amounts (Pao 1979). HANES found vitamin A intake to be below standard only among black females twelve to fourteen years of age in the high-income group, and black females aged fifteen to seventeen in the low-income group (Hodges and Krehl 1965). In addition, the proportion of adolescents with intakes below standard was high, reaching 70 percent in females fifteen to seventeen years of age. In general higher proportions of females had substandard vitamin A intake.

The standards used in biochemical determinations of serum vitamin A necessitate cautious interpretation. However, there was no indication of a potential nutritional deficiency problem in adolescents (U.S. Department of Health, Education, and Welfare 1974).

Vitamin C intake for adolescents was above recommended intakes, according to NFCS data (Pao 1979). The mean vitamin C intakes of the adolescent group in HANES were above standard, although for some adolescents vitamin C intake was low; 49 percent of females and 40 percent of males in the twelve to seventeen age group had below-standard intakes. Biochemical data have not yet been released (U.S. Department of Health, Education, and Welfare 1974). Clinical examinations revealed that bleeding, swollen gums—a sign of moderate deficiency—were found in adolescents, especially among blacks (Lowenstein 1976). Until vitamin C nutritional status is analyzed using all the parameters, it will be difficult to distinguish between a possible vitamin C deficiency and oral hygiene problems. The HANES standard for vitamin C, however, does reflect the higher levels in the most recent 1979 RDAs, while the NCFS survey uses the 1974 lower standard (Pao 1979, Institute of Medicine 1979).

In regard to *B vitamins*, NFCS reported that adolescent mean intakes of thiamin and riboflavin met recommendations (Pao 1979). HANES found mean thiamin and riboflavin intakes generally above standard. The proportion of adolescents below standard was small (Department of Health, Education, and Welfare 1979b). Biochemical results have not yet been released (Department of Health, Education, and Welfare 1974). Vitamin B-6 mean intake, reported by NFCS, was low among females fifteen years and older. In view of the questionable reliability of food composition data on B-6, this conclusion is made cautiously. Additional reports on other B vitamins are not available at this time.

Minerals. Overall *calcium* intakes were lower in 1965 than in 1978, according to NFCS (Pao 1979). Adolescent males had the highest calcium intake of all groups; nine- to eleven-year-olds and twelve- to fourteen-year-olds had the highest intakes among females. The mean intake of adolescent males met recommended amounts, but that of females did not (Pao 1979). HANES reported that mean calcium intake met or exceeded standards for all adolescents. The proportion of males with intakes below standard was relatively low (16 to 18 percent). Among females twelve to seventeen years old, high proportions of blacks (50 percent) and of whites (33 percent) had intakes below standard (Department of Health, Education, and Welfare 1979b). Biochemical and clinical assessments of calcium will reveal more information on the possible consequences of these data.

NFCS reported mean *iron* intake below RDAs for both males and females (Pao 1979). According to HANES, black males fifteen to seventeen years old in all income groups and white males fifteen to nineteen years old in the low-income group had mean intakes below dietary standards. Some 42 to 68 percent of adolescent girls aged twelve to seventeen had mean iron intakes that were below standard; the proportion of males with below-standard intakes reached 77 percent among blacks aged twelve to nineteen years (U.S. Department of Health, Education, and Welfare 1979b).

Findings on biochemical indices of iron status, including hemoglobin, serum iron, and percent transferrin saturation do not necessarily indicate poor iron nutrition as dietary intake data indicate (U.S. Department of Health, Education, and Welfare 1979d). Further interpretation of these data is needed.

To summarize, the data in HANES and NFCS suggest the following observations about the dietary intake of calories, vitamins, minerals, and iron by adolescents:

1. Caloric intake peaks at the time of the adolescent growth spurt but is below standard for this period.
2. Protein intake is generally adequate but below the recommended amount for many females.
3. Vitamin A intake, although generally adequate, is below the recommended amount for many females.
4. Vitamin C intake is adequate, but a substantial minority of adolescents have intakes below standard.
5. Thiamin and riboflavin intake is adequate; vitamin B-6 may be a concern for females over fifteen years of age.
6. Calcium intake is generally adequate but below standard for a substantial proportion of females.
7. Iron intake is below standard for females and for a large proportion of males, particularly blacks.

All biochemical, clinical, and anthropometric measurements have not been reported, nor have correlations with dietary intake been made. Additional reports will be filed on other nutrients. The total picture of nutritional status during adolescence is not yet complete. Still, these trends in dietary intake indicate directions in programming and may point to dietary lacks or excesses (Huenemann 1971).

Special Topics in Nutritional Status of Adolescents. HANES preliminary data from the *dental health* examinations revealed a high incidence of dental disease among adolescents (U.S. Department of Health, Education, and Welfare 1979a). Dietary consumption, especially sucrose, and dietary patterns, especially frequency of eating, may play a part in dental disease.

Obesity may affect 20 percent or more of the adolescent population (Coates and Thoresen 1978), and may be caused by lack of physical activity rather than excess intakes of calories (Huenemann 1972, Seltzer and Mayer 1970). Whatever the cause, adolescent obesity tends to persist into adulthood (Coates and Thoresen 1978), and obese adolescents will therefore encounter increased risks of adult diseases.

Pregnancy is a period of increased nutritional need for a female of any age. In view of the rise in birth rate among adolescent girls, pregnancy during adolescence should be of special concern to those investigating nutritional status (Polley 1979). Several findings support this concern, for example, the higher incidence of low birth weight among infants born to adolescent mothers (Berg et al. 1979). Also, Marinoff and Schonholz (1972) note that successful pregnancy among adolescents is linked more closely to starting weight and total weight gain than to chronological or gynecological age.

Biological Implications of Growth and Maturation

Studies of physiological changes in adolescence suggest directions for nutrition and health education. These studies reveal both the strengths and weaknesses of this age group.

Adolescence starts with changes in hormonal activities and ends with the last stages of sex organ and physical maturation (Valadian 1971). This period of physical change is known as the adolescent growth spurt. There is controversy as to how much order exists in this growth and maturation process compared to earlier processes (Valadian 1971, Roche 1976). Difficulty arises because of the wide variation in the timing of the growth spurt. The chronological age of adolescence (twelve to nineteen) does not necessarily coincide with the age of physical and sexual maturation.

The most widely accepted measures for clinical assessment of maturational age are those developed by Tanner (1973). Females usually mature two years before males. Maturation can begin as early as nine years of age in the female, whereas maturation in the male is not likely to begin before age eleven (Valadian 1979). However, the end of adolescent growth is difficult to establish, especially in males, whose growth in stature may not be completed until after the chronological age of adolescence (Roche 1976).

This wide variation in physical maturation, both between the sexes and among individuals, makes it difficult to target educational programs toward specific age groups. Growth and maturation variations also make it difficult to establish nutritional requirements or recommendations for adolescents in terms of chronological age.

Psychological Aspects of Adolescence

Adolescence has been defined as the period of life when social, psychological, and cognitive maturation takes place (Millar 1975). Fine has divided adolescence into three developmental stages: during "early adolescence," the individual casts off childhood and enters into adolescence; "middle adolescence" is typified by strong peer group allegiances and involvement in the adolescent subculture; and "late adolescence" is marked by emergence into adulthood and establishment of adult values (Fine 1973). A person moving through adolescence is trying to establish independence, identity, self-esteem, normal relationships with peers (especially the opposite sex), and cognitive and vocational skills (Millar 1975, Fine 1973). The adolescent also has the major psychological task of adjusting to physical changes in appearance and dealing with a new body image. The difficulty of this task is augmented by the great variation in the timing of maturation—one's own may not match that of one's peers (Institute of Medicine 1979). In fact, being an early or late maturer can have considerable and perhaps lasting effects on an individual's behavior (Tanner 1973).

In this period of enormous physical, psychological, and emotional change, the school environment plays a large part. Knowledge and job skills for adult life are acquired in school. Here, too, adolescents find the highly prized peer group relationships and the symbols of the adolescent subculture, such as dress, music, language, and even food. There is some alienation or rejection of adults, especially parents, and of adult values as the adolescent establishes a sense of identity and self-esteem.

To reach maturity and establish a sense of identity, adolescents act out and experiment with adult roles (Erikson 1963). In fact, behavioral experimentation is usually the method the adolescent uses to progress from childhood to adulthood (Fine 1973). This experimentation includes health-related behaviors, such as nutrition and exercise habits, although these may seem secondary to experimentation in sex, drugs, and alcohol (Kovar 1978). All these behaviors can have lifelong implications for health and well-being.

To some extent, food habits can be better understood in this context of development. The adolescent values the food patterns accepted by peers, and these patterns may or may not be those of adults. Some research indicates that major changes in dietary patterns occur during adolescence and tend to persist into adulthood. At this time, the adolescent is moving into an adult role and becoming responsible for personal food choices (Institute of Medicine 1978).

The major concern that shapes food choices in early adolescence often is concern over body image. The fad dieting and dietary restrictions that many adolescent females follow in their relentless pursuit of thinness, seem psychologically motivated, and at the extreme lead to the condition known as anorexia nervosa. As Bruch described, "by controlling their eating, some feel for the first time that there is a core to their personality and that they are in touch with their feelings" (1978). Anorexia nervosa can be triggered by alarm over bodily changes during puberty, causing females in particular to interpret normal developmental changes as "fatness." The severe emaciation and malnutrition that result often make it difficult to discover the precipitating psychological issues underlying subtle patterns of interaction and expectations at home.

Body image concerns male as well as female adolescents. In Berkeley, California, researchers followed 1,000 teenagers over a period of four years, and reported the following in 1966 and 1967: "The predominant attitude of these teenagers was dissatisfaction with their weight, fatness or leanness, stature, and certain other body dimensions" (Huenemann et al. 1974). About 50 percent of the girls were extremely or "fairly" concerned about overweight. They wanted smaller hips, thighs, and/or waists. A large number of girls described themselves as fat, the number increasing as the girls grew older. Approximately 50 percent of the boys were concerned about underweight and expressed a desire for larger biceps, chest, wrists, shoulders, and forearms.

Dwyer (1979, 1973), working with other researchers in 1966, found that of 446 female senior girls, 61.4 percent reported they had dieted to lose weight at some time in their life; 37.0 percent reported they were on a reducing diet on the day questioned. Most of the girls surveyed wanted to weigh less than they did; 80 percent gave desired weights lower than reported weights. However, on the basis of triceps measure, only 15.2 percent of the senior girls were obese. All the adolescents, male and female, expressed negative feelings about one or more aspects of their physical appearance. Dwyer (1979) concluded: "Weight control programs at the high school level should be planned to stress the heterogeneous character of adolescent growth as well as to stress realistic goals for weight for obese and non-obese alike."

Nutrition educators must find ways to diffuse adolescent misconceptions. As Dwyer (1973) noted in writing about the psychosexual aspects of weight control and dieting behavior:

A great deal of confusion seems to exist in many adolescents' minds between what are attainable norms or realistic expectations and what are virtually unattainable ideals and unrealistic with respect to physical appearance. Clearly, both the feminine ideal of a slender, full-bosomed model's build and the masculine ideal of the barrel-chested, muscle-bound football halfback are realizable for only a small percentage of the population, since such body builds occur only rarely in actuality.

INTERVENTION PROGRAMS: GRADES SEVEN THROUGH TWELVE

Reports of specific nutrition education programs for grades seven through twelve are divided into two major categories: nonevaluated or subjectively evaluated education efforts and evaluated programs.

Nonevaluated Programs

Reports of nonevaluated or subjectively evaluated programs are useful in that they provide ideas for learning activities; many are recorded in such data bases as ERIC, AGRICOLA, and CAIN (Florio 1980). Without evaluative procedures, however, the teacher has no feedback on instructional success and on student progress rates and need for subsequent instruction (Cooper and Go 1976). The absence of sound evaluation also widens the knowledge gap about what approaches work best for what groups, and undermines efforts to replicate potentially successful programs (Institute of Medicine 1979).

Many curricula and teaching materials exist for use in grades seven through twelve (Cooper and Go 1976, Go 1976, Wanzek and Lindgren 1977). However, many of these are not validated for learner and teacher success; in fact, the curricula themselves lack evaluation (Cooper and Go 1976, Go 1976). In addition, many of these materials require a low skill level for mastery of concepts, that is, only the simplest knowledge concepts are taught. By their very nature, these programs omit analysis for and application to real life situations (Cooper and Go 1976).

Evaluated Programs

Intervention programs are usually evaluated on the basis of student outcomes in one or a combination of the three learning domains: cognitive (knowledge), affective (attitudes and values), and behavioral (practices). Funding, time, and expertise are limiting factors in evaluating intervention programs in the secondary schools, but these evaluations are valuable to other investigators who analyze the programs' successes and failures.

Ten programs described here not only have tried to measure student reactions but also have used innovative approaches to involve adolescents. We also describe two new programs, which are now moving out of their pilot stages, and programs specially targeted to pregnant and obese adolescents.

Knowledge gains in a high school minicourse, *Body Weight as a Health Index,* were measured in an inquiry-oriented approach. Laboratory experiments allowed students to relate energy metabolism concepts to their daily experiences. The minicourse was meant as a preventive and educational measure for nonobese students and was integrated into high school biology or chemistry classes. Statistical analyses of pre- and post-test results, in a formative evaluation of the six concepts, indicated that students learned 37 percent ($\pm$ 8 percent) of the material and that learning outcomes could be regarded as satisfactory (n = 77). Successive revisions of the course materials seemed to affect scores advantageously. However, the small amount of experimental data did not allow analytical separation of the effects of instruction and material quality on learning outcomes. A course assessment questionnaire indicated that students and teachers both had positive attitudes toward this educational approach. Shortage of class time, insufficient teacher preparedness, and technical difficulties in laboratories were identified as the most common problems (Palgi et al. 1976).

Cross-age teaching has been used as a method of motivating adolescents to increase their knowledge of nutrition (MacKenzie and Arbor 1979, Carruth and Foree 1971). In cross-age teaching, high school students learn nutrition by preparing lessons to teach to other age groups. Thus, student involvement becomes an integral part of this teaching method.

MacKenzie and Arbor (1979) tested the effect of cross-age teaching on gains in nutrition knowledge among high school students. Two experimental classes were assigned the task of teaching classes on nutrition to younger children or older adults. A nutrition unit was taught for eight class periods to both the experimental groups and a control group. The experimental groups then spent four class periods planning and implementing lessons for their respective age groups. The control group spent those four class periods reviewing the concepts through discussion, debate, films, role playing, and games. Every effort was made to use motivational techniques. A pretest revealed no significant differences in nutrition knowledge among the two groups. On a different posttest, the experimental groups scored significantly higher than the control group. The higher posttest scores of the experimental groups were attributed to cross-age teaching. Subjective evaluation by the authors reported a lack of discipline problems and increase in school attendance in the experimental groups. In addition, a marked attitude change toward the elderly, from apprehension to acceptance, was observed among the students who taught older persons.

Two studies used cartoons and comics as a way of improving nutrition knowledge and motivating high school students. Through pre- and post-tests, Carruth and Foree (1971) found that programmed instruction with visual presentation of concepts led to greater knowledge gains than the more traditional approach of "learning packets." A retention test administered six weeks after instruction revealed no statistically significant loss of knowledge in either group. Subjective evaluations by students and teachers were positive.

Mapes (1977) surveyed 281 students in New York to determine their nutrition interests and their preferences for printed resources. From a list of twelve, body image and weight control were chosen as the areas of greatest concern. Students chose the following items as appealing features of printed resources: cartoons, comics, variety of articles, quick answers, and crossword puzzles. A comic format was then used to present information on body image, fad dieting, and soft drinks to a "typical" fifteen- to seventeen-year-old. Results indicated that students aged fourteen to eighteen were better able to select the intended message in the comic from a list of five or six choices (n = 721) than were students aged eight to thirteen; 63 percent of correct responses for the intended messages were reported for the entire population sample. Additional student reactions, solicited through use of a coupon on the comic book, were favorable.

Following an eight-week mass media campaign using television, radio, and brochures, Axelson and DelCampo (1978) reported increased scores on pre- and post-tests of nutrition knowledge among both experimental and control groups of ninth graders (n = 400). Nutrition information was broadcast on those television and radio stations and during those times identified as popular by the experimental students. Control groups were located outside of this range of broadcast. The media campaign included student participation in a radio quiz contest. Brochures were distributed through the central school system after two weeks of airing the nutrition spots. The experimental group's gain in knowledge was partially obliterated, because their mean pretest score was significantly lower than that of the control group, and a regression toward the mean typically occurs after a learning period. Nevertheless, blacks in the experimental group made the greatest improvement in knowledge when compared to controls. Since the experimental group of blacks had the lowest pretest scores, this gain may be explained by the fact that they had the most to learn. Also, the black population had a larger participation rate (25 percent) than the white population (4.6 percent) in the radio contests. Two factors may have contributed to this: using one radio station with primarily black programming and featuring a black singer and black athletes in the spots. The implication here is that education programs targeted toward particular subgroups can be effective.

A twenty-hour food and nutrition minicourse for eleventh and twelfth grade biology and chemistry courses was developed and evaluated in terms of knowledge, attitude, and behavior changes of the students. In lecture/discussion sessions concurrent with laboratory experiments, students analyzed the nutrient composition of four typical U.S. meals and used these meals in a rat-feeding study to determine their effect on health. In addition, a sensory demonstration of foods by the students was used to improve awareness of ways in which the senses can affect food choices.

Two initial development trials, with the author as teacher, demonstrated the feasibility of this minicourse for high school classroom use (Picardi and Pariser 1975). After a teacher workshop, field trials were conducted with three matched experimental and three control classes from two high schools. According to the results of a knowledge test, analyzed for reliability, each experimental group showed significantly larger gains in knowledge than the corresponding control group (Picardi and Porter 1976). Of special note in this study was the use of an easily administered, fifteen-minute paired comparison test to measure nutrition-related attitudes and behavior. This technique allowed the researchers to categorize student responses systematically in order to determine how responses to selected items were interrelated.

The attitude-behavior test was divided into two sections: health concerns and food choice behavior. In the first section students checked the one of each pair of nutrition-related health problems that was their greater concern. Pre- and post-test scores changed significantly within the experimental group, but comparisons of experimentals and controls revealed no significant differences in score changes. In the section on food choice behavior students checked the one of each pair that better described how they chose foods. Significant differences were reported in some areas between experimental and control groups for different trial sections, but no commonality was observed. Reliability testing indicated that students had difficulty giving consistent answers in this section, more so than with health concerns.

Correlations among knowledge, attitudes, and behavior were low in frequency and different in each trial. For example, students who were concerned about tooth decay did not necessarily avoid choosing foods high in sugar or have a high level of knowledge about sugar.

Students gave positive ratings to the minicourse, especially those parts in which students were actively involved. Although attitudes and behavior were not affected, this may have been due to the short duration of the program or immediate administration of the posttest.

Spitze (1976) used a two-week program of games and discovery learning to improve high school students' nutrition knowledge, attitudes, and food preferences. Pre- and post-test scores were obtained on a nutrition knowledge test, a questionnaire, and selection of "the fifteen foods I'd most like to eat tomorrow if these were all I could have" from a list of eighty-four foods (n = 50). The results showed a significant knowledge gain. Attitudes toward nutrition, measured by the questionnaire, showed only a positive trend toward perceiving nutrition as an interesting subject for study. Food preference changes were not statistically significant. Anonymous letters to the teacher (the author) contained mostly favorable comments about the use of games as an educational technique.

Podell et al. (1978) taught a course in cardiovascular nutrition to tenth grade biology students. Pre- and post-test measurements were made of knowledge, attitudes, reported dietary behavior, and actual serum cholesterol and triglyceride levels. The five hours of cardiovascular education included lectures, movies, relevant reading materials, and student self-analysis of a two-day food diary for saturated fat, polyunsaturated fat, and cholesterol consumption. In addition, parents whose children were identified as above the fiftieth percentile for serum lipids were notified and advised to contact their family physician for information about diet modification.

Results from the posttest, administered seven months after completion of the course, showed significant improvements in cardiovascular nutrition knowledge; five of six parameters measuring attitude also indicated a significant positive change. (Students with a family history of elevated serum cholesterol were more likely to show positive changes in attitude.) Food frequency data, used to measure improvement in eating patterns, also reflected a marked improvement—more so among females than males and more so among students in the upper quartile of initial cholesterol levels than among those in the lower quartile.

A one-year follow-up test showed significantly higher and similar values for serum cholesterol in the experimental and matched control groups. Serum triglycerides increased somewhat, with no differences in experimental and control values.

The majority of parents interviewed three months after the program reported their children were interested in and enthusiastic about the program, with many asking for family diet changes. Most parents did not see a need for diet change unless a high cholesterol problem existed. Half the parents who had been notified of their child's high cholesterol problem had notified their physician and claimed to be instituting dietary changes.

This program was well received by students, teachers, and parents. Students learned how to follow a cholesterol-lowering diet. Whether reported attitude and diet changes reflected actual changes in behavior or simply mirrored what the subject presumed the examiner wanted to hear is not known. Indications that the greatest changes in knowledge, attitude, and behavior occurred among those students in the upper quartile of serum cholesterol levels lend support to the program's real effect. Perception of a low-risk status by many of the students and their parents probably diminished their motivation to make a dietary change.

A program of nutrition education designed to change food habits and increase the acceptability of school lunch foods was offered to fifth, seventh, and tenth grade classes (Head 1974). Evaluation was based on students' ratings of school foods, weight and nutrient content of school cafeteria plate waste, performance on cognitive tests, and dietary recall records. A one-week nutrition education workshop was given to teachers, after which they developed their own plans for nutrition education. In seventh grade nutrition was taught to health classes using conventional teaching methods and tasting parties; tenth graders in a biology course conducted rat-feeding studies and calculated the adequacy of their own diets, among other activities.

Results showed knowledge improvement in seventh graders; dietary recall data indicated improved diets, but the analysis based on Basic Four was not adequate for sound interpretation. Plate waste and food acceptability changes were not apparent in the seventh and tenth grade groups. The greatest effects of this program were measured in fifth graders, where teacher and administrative support was strongest.

The author noted that teacher attitudes and teaching techniques varied widely and were probably important factors in program success. Use of the Basic Four by secondary level teachers probably was a negative factor; this approach results in low interest among high school students, possibly because the elements of discovery, interest, and meaning are absent (Dwyer et al. 1970, Poolton 1972).

Herzog et al. (1978) offered an informal, three-week nutrition education program in a high school cafeteria. Nutrition knowledge, food consumption patterns, and plate waste were measured before and after the program. Table tents and wall posters in the cafeteria showed levels of calcium, iron, and ascorbic acid in various foods. No change was found in the pre- and post-test nutrition knowledge scores of ninth graders, and no effect of the program on food selection and/or plate waste could be detected. The short period of intervention and/or the lack of classroom follow-up could explain this program's lack of effect.

What are the long-term effects of nutrition education; if knowledge is increased, does this affect behavior? An Ohio study found no consistent association between previous enrollment in high school home economics courses and present nutritional knowledge, attitudes, and practices of high school graduates, four years after commencement (Schwartz, Dalrymple, and Vivian 1974; Schwartz 1975). In fact, knowledge of nutrition and positive attitudes toward nutrition were gained from sources other than high school home economics courses, mainly out of school.

The research findings supported relationships between nutrition knowledge and attitudes and between nutrition attitudes and practices; the correlation between knowledge and practices was not significant. The interrelationship of these factors was modeled as K <---> A <---> P; that is, attitudes mediate knowledge and practices.

New Programs

The National Dairy Council has available the first two sections of Level Four in *FOOD... Your Choice* for grades seven through ten. Four separate new strands have been pretested for use in home economics, health, science, and social studies courses. The council conducted a formative evaluation to verify the module activities, working at nine sites with a total of sixteen schools and twenty-five teachers. Following data gathering and revision of curricular materials, the council returned to the field for a follow-up achievement study of home economics and health. An achievement test (knowledge based) is being designed for use with this level (as was done with Levels One through Three in *FOOD... Your Choice*). Short evaluation sections are also included in each unit. A summative evaluation is planned for 1981. This sequence of planning for and engagement in evaluation provides a model for similar efforts (Brun 1980).

The American Health Foundation has carefully piloted its *Know Your Body* program in the greater metropolitan New York area. Focusing on disease prevention, this program involves students and teachers in a series of activities initiated by a fifty-two-item survey to evaluate student knowledge in the areas of smoking, nutrition, and blood pressure. The results of this health knowledge questionnaire provide baseline information that can be used to measure changes in students' level of knowledge.

Teachers are asked prior to and during the program to complete questionnaires on the kind of classroom instruction and supplemental resources they use. Students with parental consent participate in a health-screening program that includes individual confidential reports on blood pressure, blood glucose, serum cholesterol, hematocrit, height, weight, and results of a physical fitness test that measures heart response to challenging exercise. Workshops help the teacher plan learning activities in the following areas: risk factors, smoking, nutrition principles and prevention, fat in the diet, blood pressure, physical fitness/exercises, and primary cancer prevention. Level I of the curriculum is for the sixth through eighth grades; Level II, for the ninth and tenth grades.

The overall goal of this program of risk factor prevention is to increase health knowledge and identify relationships between risk factors and personal health behavior. The curriculum strives to help students accept responsibility for their own health and practice good health habits. "Evaluation results from the *Know Your Body* program suggest that active participation by students in program activities leads to greater motivation for behavior change than if such involvement is absent" (Institute of Medicine 1979). Students have the opportunity to keep their health record and update it annually to evaluate changes in their risk factor levels.

Programs for Special Groups

Pregnancy. In addition to being a health risk, pregnancy is a major cause of school dropout among females (Polley 1979, Berg et al. 1979, Stine and Kelley 1970). Here begins a vicious cycle of inadequate health and nutrition; poor job opportunities; depressed economic status; dependence on welfare; alienation and isolation from friends, family, and society; repeat pregnancies; and, if married, likelihood of divorce (Polley 1979; Edwards, Steinman, and Hakanson 1977; Levenson et al. 1979). Pregnancy and motherhood expose adolescents to increased emotional, psychological, and developmental stresses which can affect the health and nutrition status of both mother and child (Levenson et al. 1979, Dohrmann 1979). Schools have the potential to provide quality care and education for pregnant adolescents while keeping these students in school. In-school programs have improved pregnancy outcomes by encouraging more healthful behavior during pregnancy (Stine and Kelley 1970).

The ability of schools to keep pregnant adolescents in school is complex, for pregnancy is not the only factor in high school attrition (Chilman 1979). Females show a higher dropout rate between the second and fourth years of high school than males. In addition, the proportion of females who drop out is higher than the proportion who give birth to children either within or outside of marriage during high school. Chilman noted that some of the characteristics which are typical of female high school dropouts also pertain to pregnant adolescents.

Three studies reported on an in-school health service clinic in St. Paul, Minnesota (Berg et al. 1979; Edwards, Steinman, and Hakanson 1977; Alton 1979). Berg's group compared maternity patients receiving care in an in-school program with a group enrolled in an out-of-school clinic. The study group initiated care earlier; had more prenatal visits; and experienced fewer obstetrical complications, delivery complications, and low birth weight infants than the comparison group. Since high-risk factors have been attributed largely to inadequate prenatal care (Marinoff and Schonholz 1972), these St. Paul findings are important. Since both the in-school and out-of-school groups had high incidences of nutritional problems, especially anemia, the nutrition education component of this program (not described) needed special emphasis.

In an associated study Edwards, Steinman, and Hakanson (1977) reported the results of a comprehensive high school health clinic which offered health care for pregnant adolescents and day care for infants of adolescent mothers attending school. A thirteen-week prenatal education program was part of this project. No low birth weights or prenatal deaths were reported among the 38 adolescents in the clinic. Early initiation of care, decreased rate of postpartum dropout, and a decreased rate of repeat pregnancies also were reported.

Other in-school programs with a strong nutrition component report low incidences of prematurity and low birth weight, earlier and more consistent prenatal care, and high completion rates for high school (Schwartz et al. 1974, Stine and Kelley 1970, Levenson et al. 1979). Two programs (Stine and Kelley 1970, Dohrmann 1978) were in special schools for mothers within the public school system. Day care services and/or instruction in parenting skills can help adolescent parents, whose infants are particularly susceptible to physical and developmental delay problems. Texas school districts, working with community health organizations, provided teachers to instruct adolescent mothers who had left the formal school structure (American Health Foundation 1979). Basic academic and parenting skills, including child nutrition, were taught for high school credit.

In a survey of a nonrandomly selected group of young parents, Jekel (1979) found that skills for living an independent family life were rated as their most important needs. These included driving, parenting, health care, and home economics—a wide range of skills currently taught in public school programs. Mothers who stay in school may be more mature than those who drop out and thus more capable of learning adequate nutrition (Schwartz et al. 1979). The schools have unique features that contribute to favorable pregnancy outcomes for these students. The very presence of a health clinic within a public school can increase adolescent awareness of the need for care, thereby encouraging early initiation of care (Berg et al. 1979, Stine and Kelley 1970). Programs in school also reinforce the use of medical and social services (Stine and Kelley 1970); provide emotional and psychological support (Berg et al. 1979; Stine and Kelley 1970; Edwards, Steinman, and Hakanson 1977); and counsel and educate in the varied areas of parenting, family planning, job skills, and proper health and nutrition practices (Polley 1979; Berg et al. 1979; Stine and Kelley 1970; Edwards, Steinman, and Hakanson 1977; Dohrmann 1979; Alton 1979). Other benefits to adolescents receiving pre- and post-natal care and education in school include improved nutrition through school lunch, an opportunity to supplement their calcium intake, and regular and structured hours for activity and eating (Schwartz, Dalrymple, and Vivian 1974).

Not every school can provide comprehensive health care, but through cooperation and coordination between administration and faculty and among faculty, many educational and even noneducational services can be provided. The varied curricula of public high schools, in contrast to specialized pregnancy schools, enable students to learn many life skills not directly related to pregnancy and parenting. In light of the importance of peer group allegiances in adolescent development (Fine 1973) and the detrimental effect of isolation on pregnant adolescents, it seems most advantageous for the pregnant adolescent to stay in the "mainstream of adolescent growth" (Berg et al. 1979).

In designing approaches for counseling pregnant girls, Hatcher (1973, 1976) considered developmental stages and what is known about chronological versus developmental age. Hatcher tested the theory that if pregnant adolescents were divided into the appropriate developmental groupings, one could forecast both their concerns and the appropriate counseling strategies to use. She observed that the same level of personality functioning found in each stage of adolescence prevails in the pregnancy experience and also after abortion. This type of approach may be useful in public schools.

Obesity. In-school programs attempting to decrease adiposity (fatness) in adolescents included nutrition education, exercise, psychological support, and reinforcement of program components in the home. Exercise programs emphasized self-improvement rather than competition. Nutrition education emphasized wise food selection rather than prescribing low-calorie diets. In part, diets were avoided because of possible unknown effects of caloric restriction during growth. Instead, the major emphasis was placed on decreasing body fat.

A ten-month program conducted by Seltzer and Mayer (1970) resulted in a greater slowing of the growth of triceps skinfold in treatment than in control subjects, although this finding was statistically significant only in male elementary school students. Following eighteen months of observation, Christakis et al. (1966) reported a decrease in percent overweight of experimental versus control groups (as indicated by skinfold thicknesses). The research-ers also noted an improvement in performance scores on two of five physical fitness tests and a decrease in overall weight gain in ex-perimental versus control groups. Both of these studies found trends toward accelerated obesity in the control groups of obese adolescents.

Only Seltzer and Mayer have reported follow-up data (1970). Three years after termination of the program (due to funding cut-backs) all effects of the program were eliminated, lending support to the hypothesis that such programs can be effective in the long term only when the program is sustained (Coates and Thoresen 1978).

These types of in-school programs have demonstrated positive behavioral effects and have many advantages; for example, they can be taught to large numbers of persons in existing institutions (Seltzer and Mayer 1970). Although much of the success of these programs depends on individual student motivation, collaboration of community professionals, school personnel (both administrators and faculty), and parents can result in successful implementation given appropriate facilities both at home and in school (Seltzer and Mayer 1970).

Shortcomings and Benefits of Programs

What can one say overall about the evaluated programs to date? Some shortcomings and benefits can be enumerated that may help future investigators.

One shortcoming of the evaluations is that they measure gains in nutrition knowledge of groups in short-term programs without follow-up to determine retention and/or changes in attitudes and behaviors in regard to foods and nutrition.

Another shortcoming is inadequate reporting of program materials, which makes it difficult to evaluate the type of educa-tional approach used. In addition, until recently, journals which contain such reports have not instituted reviews for program and evaluation design.

A third shortcoming concerns methodology. The methods for collecting information on food intake, such as the twenty-four-hour recall, although currently being evaluated, raise questions of validity and reliability. Inability to eliminate self-reporting bias and to account for habitual food patterns necessitates cautious interpretation of data collected by such methods.

Methodologies for implementation of programs intended to change behavior and attitudes are still in an early state of development. Further, lack of information on how knowledge, attitudes, and behavior interrelate and are mediated by each other hampers results. Similar methodological problems exist with data collection on attitude and behavioral change.

In a related area, Green (1977) identified some dilemmas faced by health education researchers: rigor versus significance, internal versus external validity, and experimental versus placebo effects, to name a few. The dilemma of long- versus short-term evaluation perhaps is the most acute. "Most of the benefits of health education are time dependent. . . . Some effects of health education are immediate and temporary, others are slower in developing but longer lasting. The so-called "sleeper effect' in much behavior change occurs when the audience must go through a process of attitude change between the educational exposure and the actual change in behavior that yields the health benefits." Seldom do researchers have the opportunity to conduct long-term, much less longitudinal, studies which would give hard data on the sleeper effect. The dilemma of funding exacerbates this problem. Green noted that "it is a tragic fact of much health education funding that the budget is below the minimum required to obtain a desired effect."

Another research problem is poor targeting of the message. Traditionally school interventions have attempted to teach general classes about health behavior. What is missing is research that compares the use of highly targeted health messages directed toward high-risk populations within the schools with the more broad-based approach.

It must be noted that some of the programs we have described have attempted to deal with these problems of evaluation. In fact, innovative educational approaches for adolescents have been tested with some promising results. This research suggests productive directions for program and evaluation design in adolescent nutrition education.

HEALTH CONCERNS OF ADOLESCENTS IN A CHANGING LIFE-STYLE

Adolescents account for 19 percent of the U.S. population. This sizable group of youth is characterized by high accident and suicide rates and increasing use of drugs, alcohol, and cigarettes. Both the rising number and the young age of pregnant adolescents have been of particular concern to health and education professionals because of the multifaceted problems faced by these school-age parents, not least of which is the high incidence of low birth weight babies.

A new approach has emerged in the area of adolescent health care. A surge of interest by the medical profession in adolescent medicine has been accompanied by the treatment of adolescents in clinical counseling as individuals worthy of time, attention, and sincerity. A parallel trend in the nutritional sciences is for educators to solicit the interests and opinions of youth as a basis for programming. Several investigators have asked adolescents to rank their top health concerns (Brunswick 1969; Sternlieb and Munan 1972; Kirk, Hamrick, and McAfee 1975), and some educators have narrowed the questioning to specific nutritional concerns (Mapes 1977; Dwyer, Feldman, and Mayer 1970). Weight loss and dieting were top concerns, as well as questions about the proper foods to eat, the value of snacking, and the relationship of food to acne. Pregnancy and alcohol also were cited as topics of special interest to adolescents.

Programming based on the concerns of the target group may produce positive results. At the 1974 Nutrition Education Conference at Penn State, Paul Fine reported: "The most important general rule that we have found for giving guidance to successful communication is that communication must enter people's lives where they are—that the communication and the product must fit the lifestyles and the needs of the consumers as they are, not as we might wish them to be." A prime example is food waste, a topic which, in an environmental context, may become a backdoor to nutrition education. Food waste has normally been a high priority only for school lunch managers and parents. When youth were encouraged to take a social studies approach, their concern for air, water, and soil pollution led to active investigation. Harrison, Rathje, and Hughes (1975) turned both university and secondary students in Tucson, Arizona, into active garbage researchers. Harrison, Mapes, and Rathje (1976) reported further evidence of keen interest in nutrition among youth throughout the United States.

Based on the health concerns expressed by high school students, who placed nutrition quite low on the list, Kirk and Hamrick (1975, 1977) integrated nutrition education into the higher priority health interests, including sex education and preparation for marriage; drugs, smoking, and alcohol; social relations; venereal diseases; school and teacher indifference to students; boy-girl relations; and understanding oneself. Such attempts to reach students by addressing their concerns can provide an effective means of teaching nutrition education.

SUMMARY

In order to institute more effective nutrition education programs for the adolescent population, continuing and increased efforts are needed in three major areas.

Increase the base of data which verify the nutrition needs and status of adolescents. Longitudinal studies are needed to specify nutritional requirements during adolescent growth and development. HANES data should be expanded for longitudinal analysis, and the nutrient needs of adolescents should be better defined. Further research is required into the physiological mechanisms involving nutrients, such as enzyme systems, energy efficiency, growth, and maturation, and into the adequacy of adolescents' diets in relation to their needs.

Utilize learning strategies matched to adolescent needs, concerns, and American life-style. The educational approaches being used in nutrition education programs for adolescents often are not matched to the needs of adolescents, especially in terms of psychological development. Yet the school setting can be used to stimulate learning. Several specific recommendations should be considered in this respect.

First, encourage student participation in learning. The discovery method of teaching nutrition has been used successfully in many intervention activities reported in the last two years. Nutritionists are beginning to capitalize on one of the basic principles of learning: "Any information will affect a person's behavior only in the degree to which he has discovered its personal meaning for him" (Combs, Avila, and Purkey 1978).

Second, institute a redirected fitness program for all youth. One of the contributing causes of obesity is lack of physical activity. Most school efforts are directed toward the 5 percent of students who are athletes (Millar 1975). With the emergence of community facilities for adults and families, a new trend may be emerging. For example, over 300 exercise trails are now in use throughout the country, and 200 more are planned (Blumenthal 1979). A new, individualized approach to physical education, whereby all students participate according to their own ability and speed (Reed 1979) should facilitate a parallel approach to activities focused on food and nutrition.

Third, address the concerns of students, including obesity, pregnancy, the relationship of diet to drugs and alcohol, and the environment. Adolescents need to be treated as adolescents, not as adults or as children, and programming should be geared toward what the adolescent wants to know about nutrition. Some educators have attempted to do this (Mapes 1977; Kirk, Hamrick, and McAfee 1975). Innovative approaches which capitalize on adolescent developmental phases can turn behavioral experimentation and self-discovery into positive, self-enhancing health behavior and can reinforce existing positive behaviors.

Fourth, coordinate efforts among those involved in adolescent health and nutrition. People involved with the nutrition of adolescents often work in isolation, although on parallel tracks. The task of promoting nutritional health among adolescents is complex and requires a multifaceted approach, utilizing the coordinated efforts of health professionals, nutrition researchers, nutrition educators, school administrators and faculty, families, and the adolescents themselves. It is vital that the total environment of adolescents be considered in nutrition education.

Fifth, recognize the societal influences on health behavior and help students cope with them. The adolescent frequently receives mixed messages from adults in regard to diet and nutrition. Many Americans pay lip service to positive health values, including eating properly, but do not adopt corresponding behaviors. An example is the increasing concern over the nutritional value of foods in vending machines, accompanied by the continuing and increasing use of these vending machines in schools.

Society also influences health behavior through social conditioning. An adolescent (or adult) body image problem is not initiated in isolation, but is influenced by subjective impressions of body image norms dictated by society. Efforts to reconcile one's own body with society's image of the "perfect body" can contribute to psychological adjustment problems ranging from anxiety and unhappiness to the life-threatening cases of anorexia nervosa.

Media campaigns are another social influence on health behavior. In attempting to sell products, many advertisements emphasize the sensual aspects of food rather than its nutritional qualities. Concentration on sugar-dense foods continues to be a problem. Some nutritional claims made in advertising are so questionable that the Federal Trade Commission has been formulating standards for use in making and monitoring food claims.

Social influences and conditioning cannot be ignored in the development and implementation of nutrition education programs. Health and nutrition behaviors are not willfully or consciously chosen by an individual but rather emerge as a result of many influences.

Finally, help students take more responsibility for their health and their diet. We cannot assume that if people know what is healthy they will behave in a manner which will enhance their health. Baker and Dietz reminded us that the "emphasis on personal responsibility ignores the important role of the social, political, economic, and physical environments that largely determine behavior" (U.S. Department of Health, Education, and Welfare 1979e).

Institute evaluation methodologies appropriate to health education both in program resources and in program research. The need for evalution is great—especially in school settings where few evaluated programs are reported. Reporting should be encouraged, since insufficient and incomplete reporting decreases the opportunity for replication.

In addition, the timing of educational intervention programs needs to be studied. This problem is twofold: first, most evaluated programs have been short-term efforts and have been evaluated only immediately after implementation. Although curricula for adolescents have been developed, comprehensive evaluations showing effects on knowledge, attitudes, and behavior over time need to be done. Second, the long-term effects of short-period intervention studies need to be examined.

More knowledge is needed in regard to the appropriate age for initiation of nutrition education programs. It is not known whether a program introduced in early adolescence (twelve to thirteen years of age) can be effective in promoting health and nutrition-enhancing behaviors or whether such programs need to be started earlier. We also do not know how much reinforcement is necessary, for as Green (1977) notes, "reinforcement is as important to education as booster shots are to sustained immunization."

Many of the same suggestions were made at the Conference on Adolescent Behavior and Health (Institute of Medicine 1979). Workshop participants identified four factors critical to the design of effective school-based education programs for adolescents: (1) a developmental perspective, (2) encouragement of individual responsibility, (3) adolescent involvement, and (4) use of peer influence.

Adolescents must be treated as individuals within the contexts of their own environments and life-styles—a fact we have long known but have often failed to heed in designing effective, school-based programs.

BIBLIOGRAPHY

Alton, I.R. 1979. Nutrition Services for Pregnant Adolescents Within a Public High School. *J. Am. Dietet. Assoc.* 74:667.

American Health Foundation. 1979. *Know Your Body: Teacher's Guide.* New York:American Health Foundation.

Axelson, J., and DelCampo, D.S. 1978. Improving Teenagers' Nutrition Knowledge Through the Mass Media. *J. Nutr. Educ.* 10:30.

Berg, M. et al. 1979. Prenatal Care for Pregnant Adolescents in a Public High School. *J. Sch. Health* 49:32.

Blumenthal, D. 1979. Warming Up to the Challenge of Exercise Trails. *New York Times,* April 22.

Bruch, H. 1978. *Anorexia Nervosa: The Golden Cage.* Cambridge, Mass.: Harvard University Press.

Brun, J. 1980. Personal conversation. National Dairy Council, Rosemont, Illinois.

Brunswick, A.F. 1969. Health Needs of Adolescents: How the Adolescent Sees Them. *Am. J. Pub. Health* 59:1730.

Carruth, B.R., and Foree, S.B. 1971. Cartoon Approach to Nutrition Education. *J. Nutr. Educ.* 3:57.

Chilman, C.S. 1979. Adolescent Sexuality in Changing American Society: Social and Psychological Perspectives. DHEW Pub. no. (NIH) 79-1426.

Christakis, G. et al. 1966. Effect of a Combined Nutrition Education and Physical Fitness Program on the Weight Status of Obese High School Boys. *Federation Proc.* 25:15.

Coates, T.J., and C.E. Thoresen. 1978. Treating Obesity in Children and Adolescents: A Review. *Am. J. Pub. Health* 68:143.

Combs, A.W.; Avila, D.L.; and Purkey, W.M. 1978. *Helping Relationships.* Boston: Allyn & Bacon.

Cooper, K.A., and Go, C.E. 1976. Analysis of Nutrition Curriculum Guides at the K–12 Level. *J. Nutr. Educ.* 8:62.

Dohrmann, H. 1979. Nutrition Education in the Santa Anna Teen Mother Program. *J. Am. Dietet. Assoc.* 74:665.

Dwyer, J. 1973. Psychosexual Aspects of Weight Control and Dieting Behavior in Adolescents. *Medical Aspects of Human Sexuality* (March): 82–114.

Dwyer, J. et al. 1979. Adolescent Attitudes Toward Weight and Appearance. *J. Nutr. Educ.* 1:14–19.

Dwyer, J.; Feldman, J.J.; and Mayer, J. 1970. Nutritional Literacy of High School Students. *J. Nutr. Educ.* 2:59.

Edwards, L.E.; Steinman, M.E.; and Hakanson, E.Y. 1977. An Experimental Comprehensive High School Clinic. *Am. J. Pub. Health* 67:765.

Erikson, E.H. 1963. *Childhood and Society.* New York: W.W. Norton and Company.

Fine, L.L. 1973. What's a Normal Adolescent? *Clinical Pediatrics* 12:1.

Fine, P. 1974. Social Scientists Look at Nutrition Education. Nourishment vs. Nutrition: The Housewife's Dilemma. Proceedings of the Nutrition Education Conference, Pennsylvania State University, July 21–24, pp. 37–55.

Florio, J. 1980. Personal conversation. New York State Education Department, Educational Systems Information Service.

Go, C. 1976. An Analysis of Selected Curriculum Guides Used for Nutrition Education in Grades K–12. Berkeley: Society for Nutrition Education.

Green, L.W. 1977. Evaluation and Measurement: Some Dilemmas for Health Education. *Am. J. Public Health* 78:155.

Hama, M.Y. 1979. Changes in Nutrient Levels and Foods Used by Households in the United States, Spring 1965 and 1977. Paper presented to the 1980 Agricultural Outlook Conference, Washington, D.C., November 6.

Hatcher, S.L. 1973. The Adolescent Experience of Pregnancy and Abortion: A Developmental Analysis. *J. Youth and Adolescence* 2, no. 1.

———. 1976. Understanding Adolescent Pregnancy and Abortion. *Primary Care* 3:407.

Harrison, G.G.; Mapes, M.C.; and Rathje, W.L. 1976. Trash Tells a Tale: School Studies of Food Waste as a Tool for Nutrition Education. *Illinois Teacher* 14:298.

Harrison, G.; Rathje, W.L.; and Hughes, W.W. 1975. Food Waste Behavior in an Urban Population. *J. Nutr. Educ.* 7:13.

Head, M.K. 1974. A Nutrition Education Program at Three Grade Levels. *J. Nutr. Educ.* 6:56.

Hegsted, D.M. 1976. Current Knowledge of Energy, Fat, Protein, and Amino Acid Needs. In *Nutrient Requirements in Adolescence,* ed. J.I. McKigney and H.N. Munro. Cambridge, Mass.: MIT Press.

Herzog, L.J. 1978. The Effects of an Informal Nutrition Education Approach Conducted in Conjunction with a High School Lunch Program in Two Northern New Jersey Schools. Master's thesis, Rutgers University.

Herzog, L.J. et al. 1978. Evaluation of an Informal Nutrition Education Approach in a High School Lunch Program. *School Food Service Res. Rev.* 2:102.

Hodges, R.E. 1976. Vitamin and Mineral Requirements in Adolescence. In *Nutrient Requirements in Adolescence,* ed. J.I. McKigney and H.N. Munro. Cambridge, Mass.: MIT Press.

Hodges, R.E., and Krehl, W.A. 1965. Nutritional Status of Teenagers in Iowa. *Am. J. Clin. Nut.* 17:200.

Huenemann, R.L. 1971. A Review of Teenage Nutrition in the United States. In *Proceedings of National Nutrition Education Conference.* Misc. Pub. no. 1254:37. Washington, D.C.: U.S. Department of Agriculture.

————. 1972. Food Habits of Obese and Nonobese Adolescents. *Postgraduate Medicine* (May): 99.

Huenemann, R.L. et al. 1968 Food and Eating Practices of Teenagers. *J. Am. Dietet. Assoc.* 53:17.

————. 1974. *Teenage Nutrition and Physique.* Springfield, Illinois: Charles C. Thomas.

Institute of Medicine, National Academy of Sciences. 1979. Conference on Adolescent Behavior and Health, Washington, D.C., October.

Jekel, J.F., and Forbush, J.B. 1979. Service Needs of Adolescent Parents. *J. Sch. Health* 49:527.

Kirk, R.H., and Hamrick, M.H. 1977. *Focus on Health and Nutrition.* A Comprehensive Health Education Curriculum Guide for Grades 9–12. Rosemont, Illinois: National Dairy Council.

Kirk, R.H.; Hamrick, M.; and McAfee, D.C. 1975. Nutrition in Health Instruction: The Tennessee Health Education Project. *J. Nutr. Educ.* 7:68.

Kovar, M.G. 1978. Adolescent Health Status and Health Related Behavior. In *Conference on Adolescent Behavior and Health.* Washington, D.C.: National Academy of Sciences, Institute of Medicine.

Levenson, P. et al. 1979. A Comprehensive Interactional Model for Health Education Delivery to Teenage Mothers. *J. Sch. Health* 49:393.

Leverton, R.M. 1968. The Paradox of Teenage Nutrition. *J. Am. Dietet. Assoc.* 53:13.

Lowenstein, F.W. 1976. Preliminary Clinical and Anthropometric Findings from the First Health and Nutrition Examination Survey, USA, 1971–1972. *Am. J. Clinical Nutr.* 29:918–927.

MacKenzie, L., and Arbor, E. 1979. Cross-Age Teaching—An Important Concept for Nutrition Education. *J. Nutr. Educ.* 11:138.

Mapes, M.C. 1977. Gulp—An Alternate Method for Reaching Teens. *J. Nutr. Educ.* 9:12.

Marinoff, S.C., and Schonholz, D.H. 1972. Adolescent Pregnancy. *Pediatric Clinics of North America* 19:795.

McKigney, J.I., and Munro, H.N. 1976. *Nutrient Requirements in Adolescence.* Cambridge, Mass.: MIT Press.

Millar, H.E.C. 1975. Approaches to Adolescent Health Care in the 1970s. DHEW (HSA) Pub. no. 76–5014.

Mueller, J.F. 1976. Current Recommended Dietary Allowances for Adolescents. In *Nutrient Requirements in Adolescence,* J.I. McKigney and H.N. Munro. Cambridge, Mass.: MIT Press.

Palgi, A. et al. 1976. Body Weight as a Health Index: A Minicourse in Nutrition. *J. Nutr. Educ.* 8:126.

Pao, E.M. 1979. Nutrient Consumption Patterns of Individuals in 1977 and 1965. Paper presented at the 1980 Agricultural Outlook Conference, Washington, D.C., November 6.

Picardi, S.M., and Pariser, E.R. 1975. Food and Nutrition Minicourse for 11th and 12th Grades. *J. Nutr. Educ.* 7:25.

Picardi, S.M., and Porter, D.P. 1976. Multidimensional Evaluation of a Food and Nutrition Minicourse. *J. Nutr. Educ.* 8:162.

Podell, R.N. et al. 1978. Evaluation of the Effectiveness of a High School Course in Cardiovascular Nutrition. *Am. J. Public Health* 68:573.

Polley, M.J. 1979. Teen Mothers: A Status Report. *J. School Health* 8:466.

Poolton, M.A. 1972. Predicting Application of Nutrition Education. *J. Nutr. Educ.* 4:110.

Reed, S. 1979. The New Phys Ed Benefits Everyone. *New York Times,* April 22.

Roche, A.F. 1976. Some Aspects of Adolescent Growth and Maturation. In *Nutrient Requirements in Adolescence,* ed. J.I. McKigney and H.N. Munro. Cambridge, Mass.: MIT Press.

Schwartz, N.E. 1975. Nutritional Knowledge, Attitudes and Practices of High School Graduates. *J. Am. Dietet. Assoc.* 66:28.

Schwartz, N.E.; Dalrymple, J.I.; and Vivian, V.M. 1974. High School Nutrition Education: How Effective Is It? *J. Home Econ.* 66:16.

Seltzer, C.C., and Mayer, J. 1970. An Effective Weight Control Program in a Public School System. *Am. J. Public Health* 60:679.

Shoup, E.W. 1975. Teens Teach Children Nutrition. *J. Nutr. Educ.* 7:107.

Spitze, H.T. 1976. Curriculum Materials and Nutrition Learning at the High School Level. *J. Nutr. Educ.* 8:59.

Sternlieb, J.J., and Munan, L. 1972. A Survey of Health Problems, Practices, and Needs of Youth. *Pediatrics* 49:177.

Stine, O.C., and Kelley, E.B. 1970. Evaluation of a School for Young Mothers. *Pediatrics* 46:581.

Tanner, J.M. 1973. Growing Up. *Scientific American* 35.

U.S. Department of Health, Education, and Welfare. 1972. Ten-State Nutrition Survey. DHEW Pub. no. (HSM) 73–8704.

———. 1974. Preliminary Findings of the First Health and Nutrition Examination Survey, United States, 1971–1972. Dietary Intake and Biochemical Findings. DHEW Pub. no. (HRA) 74–1219–1.

———. 1976. Plan and Operations of the Health and Nutrition Examination Survey, United States, 1971–1973. DHEW Pub. no. (HRA) 76–1310.

———. 1979a. Basic Data for Dental Examination Findings of Persons 1–74 Years, United States, 1971–1974. DHEW Pub. no. (PHS) 79–1662.

———. 1979b. Caloric and Selected Nutrient Values for Persons 1–74 Years of Age: First Health and Nutrition Examination Survey, United States, 1971–1974. DHEW Pub. no. (PHS) 79–1657.

———. 1979c. Dietary Intake Source Data, United States, 1971–1974. DHEW Pub. no. (PHS) 79–1221.

———. 1979d. Hemoglobin and Selected Iron-Related Findings of Persons 1–74 Years of Age: United States, 1971–1974. Advanced Data 46 (January 26).

——— 1979e. Institute of Medicine, National Academy of Sciences. Healthy People: The Surgeon General's Report on Health Promotion and Disease Prevention. DHEW (PHS) Pub. no. 79–55071 –A.

Valadian, I. 1971. The Adolescent—His Growth and Development. In *Proceedings of the National Nutrition Education Conference.* Misc. Pub. no. 1254: 21. Washington, D.C.: U.S. Department of Agriculture.

Wanzek, C.S., and Lindgren, M.J. 1977. *The Chicago Nutrition Association Publications List, 1977.* Chicago: Kraft, Inc.

Wharton, M.A. 1963. Nutritive Intake of Adolescents. *J. Am. Dietet. Assoc.* 42:306.

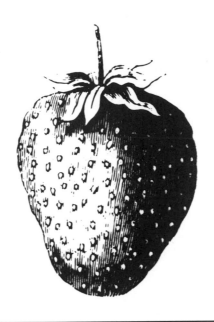

APPENDICES

APPENDIX 1: PRESCHOOL NUTRITION EDUCATION MATERIALS AND CURRICULA

Nutrition education curricula for preschoolers have been developed by university nutrition departments and by early childhood education departments, teachers, nutritionists, and parents. They usually are formatted as guides to activities, curricula, and cookbooks. Materials in this section have as the target audience the preschooler, age two to five years, not kindergarteners.

In addition to a descriptive outline, we also provide a nutritional critique based on the following criteria:

The goal(s) should address current nutrition and health issues.

Activities should use food to teach nutrition in addition to other subject areas.

Food choices and recipe selections should be consistent with the U.S. Dietary Goals; the Surgeon General's report, *Healthy People;* the recommendations of the American Society for Clinical Nutrition; and the USDA/HEW dietary guidelines.

Nutrition knowledge should be up to date and accurate.

Cookbooks

The following annotated nutrition education materials are cookbooks that provide some nutrition information, guidance, and goals for the teacher or parent.

Cool Cooking for Kids—Recipes and Nutrition for Preschool. Pat McClenahan and Ida Jaqua, Fearon Publishers Inc., Belmont, California, 1976, 170 pages. Strongly emphasizing the Basic Four, this book contains a good assortment of step-by-step recipes organized according to the need for heat. However, there are some high-sugar-content recipes included, and the nutrition information provided in the first chapter is misleading in parts.

Crunchy Bananas. Barbara Wilms, Pergrine Smith Inc., 1976, 111 pages. The first chapter integrates cooking activities into other subject areas. The seventy-six recipes are easy to prepare, appeal to children, and have some nutritional value.

Cook and Learn—A Child's Cook Book. Thelma Harms and Bec Veitch, 656 Terra California Drive #3, Walnut Creek, California, 206 pages. The first section provides hints for cooking with children, other types of learning that can be integrated with cooking, and ways of presenting recipes. The recipes are nutritious, international, single portion, and presented in a picture format children can read.

The Mother-Child Cookbook. Nancy J. Ferreira, Pacific Coast Publishers, Menlo Park, California, 73 pages. This is a guide for parents and teachers introducing children to food and food preparation and eating skills. The recipes are organized according to motor skills, age appropriateness, and food category.

Curricula

Maryland Preschool Nutrition Program

Developed: 1977–1979

From: Maryland State Educational Department
            Vocational Education
            Baltimore, Maryland

Goals: Providing children with food experiences; familiarizing children with nutrition concepts and establishing nutritionally sound food habits

Organizational Framework: First-hand experience with food and activities; Basic Four; food orientation

How to Use: For three- , four- , and five-year-olds
            Not integrated into subject matter, but activities use various modes
            Not sequenced
            Evaluation suggested through observation techniques and listening

For: Early childhood teachers and secondary students in home economics child development lab (vocational education)

Contents: 1. *Student Competencies Manual*
            10 units with information sheets, worksheets, instruction sheets

Critique
Language very sophisticated for students
Limited nutrition information provided
Resources not recommended

2. *Nutritional Instructional Materials*
   Game ideas (Concentration, Lotto, puzzles, dominoes) using Dairy Council food models

3. *5 x 8 file cards in box*
   Concept, activity, and recipe files for four food groups; some additional resources in back

   Critique:
   Not enough teacher background
   Nutritionally sound information; recipe choices ok
   Doesn't deal with nutrition and health

4. *Parent Component*
   Suggesting weekly groups plus newsletter
   Goals:
   Basic nutrition concepts (Basic Four)
   Get children to accept a variety of foods
   Improve knowledge and behavior trends
   Improve knowledge and behavior toward foods offered and thereby lay a foundation for sound nutrition and better health
   Contains background information (similar to other components), recipes, books, songs, and activities

5. Pre- and post-test manual with 60 pages of food pictures

Research: *Purpose*
To assess nutrition knowledge and attitudes
To design resource materials encouraging nutritional food choices

Design and Results
1. 58 questions similar to Peabody picture vocabulary test—validated pre-post picture test dealt with identification of foods, classification into

food groups, foods in different forms, food sources, and nutrition understanding
- After 8 weeks significant increase in cognitive scores
- After one year experimental group scores significant at .01 level
- Third-year pre-post—significant difference in total number of concepts acquired

2. Pre-post food attitudes and preferences—actual foods
- Not significant at .05
- Looking at what foods children like, choose, eat

3. Teacher evaluation
- Very enthusiastic

Early Childhood Nutrition Program

Developed: 1979 Jill Randell and Christine Olson

From: Cornell University
Distribution Center
7 Research Park
Ithaca, New York 14853

Goals: Willingness to taste a wide variety of foods, particularly fresh vegetables or fruits
Awareness of the physical and sensory characteristics of food
Knowledge that food is important for life and that a healthy body needs a number of different foods daily
Ability to distinguish between healthful and nonhealthful foods regardless of tastes
Realization of the negative consequences of consuming large amounts of sugar
Selection and enjoyment of low-sugar foods for snacks and meals
Skills and attitudes that facilitate the consumption of a nutritious diet: tasting, sitting at table, chewing food well, eating in a slow and relaxed manner, enjoying and valuing mealtime

Skills to prepare and serve food: scrubbing, mixing, tearing, and pouring

Acceptance of rules and limits about eating and cooking, and consideration of self and others

An attitude that demands verification of what is said and shown about food on television

Knowledge that people of varied cultures, upbringing, and geographic location have varied eating patterns

Ability to distinguish the sources of many different foods

Organizational Framework: Nutritional goals

How to Use: For two- to five-year-olds
Integrated into different subject areas
Not sequenced

Contents: 1. Educator's Guide: Food Experiences for Young Children (189 pages). Includes information on implementing a food and nutrition program, 4 units of nutrition activities with recipes, songs, puppet shows, stories, and resources

       2. Nutrition Activities: Preschoolers and Parents (23 pages in spirit master book or as a lightweight booklet, in English or Spanish). Contains nutrition information sheets for parents and recipes and activities for parents and children to do together in the home; tied to the four nutrition activity units in the Educator's Guide

       3. Early Childhood Educators: Nutrition Handbook (52 pages). Basic nutrition information and specific information about preschoolers' food habits, providing the background for early childhood educators conducting programs in nutrition

       4. Parents and Preschoolers: A Recipe for Good Nutrition (flip chart, 15 pages, in English and Spanish). Contains black and white photographs with suggested dialogue and discussion questions and answers. Topics for parent workshops or teacher training are: Why is Nutrition Important? How are Food Habits Formed? What Can Parents Do to Help a Child to Develop Good Eating Habits?

Nutritional Critique:
Accurate nutrition information
Addresses major nutrition concepts

Research: An evaluation of the Early Childhood Nutrition Program was completed in August 1980. Food habits and attitudes among preschool children were evaluated in programs where some teachers participated in a workshop and received the materials, some only received the materials, and some did neither.

Food—Early Choices

Developed: 1979 A nutrition learning system for early childhood

From: National Dairy Council
        Rosemont, Illinois 60018

Goals: To provide experiences that encourage wise food choices by children and the adults with whom the children interact.

1. Food is necessary for energy, growth, and health.
2. Foods have many characteristics: appearance, taste, texture, and smell.
3. Foods can be prepared in different ways.
4. All individuals need food.
5. Food can have different meanings.

Organizational Framework: Nutrition concepts

How to Use: For three- and four-year-olds and their parents
                 Sequencing is flexible after the first three activities
                 Evaluation is suggested by observation
                 Activities are integrated into different areas of child development

Contents: 1. Teacher's Guide—contains sections on using Food —Early Choices and two chapters of nutrition background information
             2. Learning Activity Cards—22 cards on objectives, procedure, materials, and additional activity ideas
             3. Resource materials—a puppet, 100 food cards, 2 decks of 36 food playing cards, puzzles, a floor mat game, a poster, a storybook, and a record

4. Parent materials—a spirit master booklet with nutrition information for parents and food-related activities that parents can do with children

Nutritional Critique:
Addresses major nutrition concepts
Accurate nutrition information
No additional nutrition resources or references are suggested
Recipes are not provided

Nutrition in a Changing World—A Curriculum for Preschool

Developed: Ellen S. Marbach, Martha Plass, Lily Usu O'Connell

From: Pennsylvania State University
Brigham Young University Press
Provo, Utah
1979, 175 pages

Goals: The curriculum includes 29 units described to help the child become:

An informed nutrition consumer appropriate to his/her age level
A person who enjoys and feels good about food
A wise snacker who thinks in terms of the total foods intake for that day
A young person who is becoming aware of the value of food (nutrients), the sources of food and the importance of amounts of food to good health and growth
A critical selector of foods who is guided by variety

Organizational Framework: Foods, nutrition goals—Basic Four

How to Use: For ages three, four, and five
29 units to be taught in sequence; 1 week per unit is suggested
All subject matter areas integrated into the nutrition activities
Evaluation includes preassessment and postassessment for each unit
Each unit also contains:
Rationale

List of material needed
Objectives
Activities, including songs, poems, puppet shows
Teacher information
Resources
Work sheets that can be duplicated
Some units contain recipes and letters to parents

Nutritional Critique:
Addresses major nutrition issues
Up-to-date and accurate nutrition information for
the teacher but limited amounts
Some food choices and activities not in keeping
with current dietary guidelines

Research: An evaluation of kindergarteners showed significant gains in knowledge (a doubling of scores) after teachers taught from the nutrition education curriculum.

Creative Food Experiences for Children

Developed: Mary Goodwin and Gerry Pollen

From: Center for Science in the Public Interest
1755 S. Street, N.W.
Washington, D.C. 20009
1974, 191 pages, $4.50

Goals: The following topics are addressed in the activities with the goal of encouraging the consumption of a variety of wholesome foods:
1. Why do we eat?
2. What is a healthy body?
3. What is in food?
4. Where does food come from?
5. Food is necessary to all living things.
6. Mealtimes
7. Food and other cultures

Organizational Framework: Food orientation

How to Use: For preschool and elementary students to be used
by parents, leaders, and teachers
122 pages of individual activities, some organized

by food type in fruit, protein, milk, etc. and
others organized by subject matter

Each activity has an objective, list of materials,
procedure

Some activities suggest resources and provide additional information to the teacher

No evaluation suggested

Additional sections provide an excellent list of
sources and resources, lunch and snack ideas and
recipes

No parent component

Nutritional Critique:

Addresses some nutrition and health issues, but
few activities are suggested to support these topics

Recipes and food choices in activities are nutritionally appropriate

Nutrition information is accurate

The Peripatetic Nutritionist

Developed: Nutritionist Education Activities in a Philadelphia
Day Care Center
Dorothy Payne Bryan, Clarence Bozeman, and Iris
Jason

From: National Urban League
1974, 44 pages

Goals: For the teacher to improve the food habits of the children
by:

Demonstrating a positive attitude toward a wide variety
of nutritionally valuable foods

Structuring experiences leading to a broader acceptance
of a wide variety of food

Applying an understanding of the interrelationships between food, health, and well-being

Organizational Framework: Nutrition education is integrated
into other subject matter areas.

How to Use: For three- , four- , and five-year-olds

9 chapters use food activities to teach and develop other curriculum areas

Evaluation suggested by looking at records (diaries, physical records, etc.) normally kept at the center

No recipes nor any substantial nutrition information provided

Ideas for parent involvement presented

Nutritional Critique:

Most activities do not have nutrition goals, although they involve food

Inadequate nutrition information for the teacher for this document to stand alone

No recipes or resources suggested

Exploring Foods with Young Children: A Recipe for Nutrition Education

Developed: Florida Department of Education
Tallahassee, Florida

Adapted from The Peripatetic Nutritionist

Humpty Dumpty Was An Egg

Developed: Joanne Ikeda and Linda Garcia
University of California
Cooperative Extension
Berkeley, California
1977, 16 pages, $1.00

Goals: To teach children that:
All living things need food and water
Food helps us grow
We get our food from plants and animals
Trying new foods can be fun

Organizational Framework: Nutrition goals

How to Use: For young children (three to eight years)
Not integrated into subject matter areas

Not sequenced

Each activity section contains behavioral objectives, list of activities, and the "how to"

Annotated resource lists, snack menus, and a few recipes

Contains suggestions for involving parents

No specific evaluation suggested except for the behavioral goals

No teacher information provided

Nutritional Critique:
Addresses major nutritional issues

No nutrition background information for teachers provided or suggested

Nutrition Education for Young Children

Developed: Project Head Start

From: U.S. Department of Health, Education, and Welfare
60 pages

Goals: To establish good food habits by:
Helping parents learn about good food, about what it does for their infants and children.
Feeding the children good food at the center.
Helping children learn about familiar foods, as well as encouraging them to taste and learn about unfamiliar foods.

Organizational Framework: Nutrition and food activities organized according to the different opportunities for the children to learn about food, meals, snack, field trips, etc.

How to Use: For Head Start children
To be used by teachers and aides
Some integration into other subject matter
Resources, parent component, and teacher information are not presented in this booklet but are available in other publications that are part of the series and in Nutrition Training Guide for Classroom Personnel in Head Start Programs,

U.S. Department of Health, Education, and Welfare, 1976

Nutritional Critique:
Of the few recipes that are presented, many have a
large amount of sugar or fat
Nutrition and health not addressed

Cooking and Eating with Children—A Way to Learn

Developed: Association for Childhood Education International
1974, 48 pages

Goals: The nutrition education goal is the establishment of good
eating practices. Cooking experiences used to teach children about
nutrition education, motor skills, social learning, etc.

Organizational Framework: Cooking experiences

How to Use: For preschool and early elementary school children
To be used by parents and teachers
Contains a guide to cooking activities and recipes
Integrated with nutrition and other subject matter

No evaluation
Not enough references
No parent component

Nutritional Critique
Most recipes have good nutritional content
Doesn't deal with nutrition and health
No general nutrition information provided

APPENDIX 2:
KINDERGARTEN THROUGH SIXTH GRADE
CURRICULA AND PROGRAMS

Berkeley Project
National Center for Health Education
School Health Education Project
901 Sneath Lane, Suite 215
San Bruno, CA 94066

enerGy thRu nUtritive Basics (GRUB)
  Rowland Unified School District
  Department of Food Services
  1830 Nogales Street
  Rowland Heights, CA 91748
Minimum Proficiency Levels for Nutrition Education in
    California Schools
  Nutrition Education and Training Program
  Child Nutrition Services Bureau
  California State Department of Education
  Sacramento, CA 95814
"Please Pass the Nutrition"
  San Jose Unified School District, Food Division
  706 West Julian
  San Jose, CA 95126
Food Education Project/Consumer Education Project
  Curriculum Research and Development Group
  College of Education, University of Hawaii and the State
    Department of Education
  Honolulu, HI 96822
FOOD . . . Your Choice
  National Dairy Council
  6300 North River Road
  Rosemont, IL 60018
Dufus Stories and *FROM THE INSIDE OUT: A Guide to Food
    and Physical Fitness*
  Learning for Life/Management Sciences for Health
  141 Tremont Street
  Boston, MA 02111
Ladybugs and Lettuce Leaves
  PROJECT OUTSIDE/INSIDE
  Somerville Public Schools
  81 Highland Avenue
  Somerville, MA 02143
Food: What's in It for You?
  Nutrition Strand Teacher Reference Guide and Minimal Per-
    formance Objectives for Health Education
  Michigan Department of Education
  Lansing, MI

Health Education Strand: Physical Dimension of Health
  Nutrition Education
  The University of the State of New York/The State Education
    Department
  Bureau of School Health Education and Services
  Albany, NY 12230
Nutrition Education in a Changing World
  The School Nutrition Curriculum Study
  Pennsylvania State University
  University Park, PA 16802
Curriculum guides available from
  Brigham Young University Press
  Provo, Utah
Nutrient Density–Nutrition Education Program
  Department of Nutrition and Food Sciences
  Utah State University
  Logan, UT 84322
Creative Food Experiences for Children
  Center for Science in the Public Interest
  1779 Church Street N.W.
  Washington, DC 20036
Nutritional Wild Edibles
  Calhoun County (West Virginia) Schools
  Vonda Gunn, Project Director
  P.O. Box 447
  Grantsville, WV 26147
Nutrition Curriculum, Kindergarten Through Sixth Grade
  Working Copy
  Child Nutrition Division
  West Virginia Department of Education
  Charleston, WV 25305

CONTRIBUTORS

Judith K. Brun, Ph.D., is Evaluation Research Associate for the National Dairy Council in Rosemont, Illinois, where she promotes and conducts research and evaluation in nutrition education. She was formerly on the faculty in the College of Education, University of Illinois, Urbana-Champaign.

Isobel Contento, Ph.D., is Associate Professor of Nutrition and Education at Teacher's College, Columbia University. She is currently on the editorial board of the *Journal of Nutrition Education.*

Judith Glotzer, B.A., a survey research specialist, is Deputy Project Director for the Abt Associates Inc. evaluation of the U.S. Department of Agriculture's Nutrition Education and Training Program.

Martha C. Mapes, B.S., M.S., is on the faculty of the Division of Nutritional Sciences at Cornell University, where she has been Division Extension Leader and youth nutrition specialist. The coauthor of *Nutrition Comes Alive,* a nutrition curriculum for K–6, she is currently working in the area of obesity, fitness, and health.

Joanne Nestor, M.C.P., was staff nutritionist for the Abt Associates Inc. evaluation of the U.S. Department of Agriculture's Nutrition Education and Training Program. She is currently a Research Associate in the International Nutrition Communications Service of Education Development Center, Inc.

Christine M. Olson, Ph.D., is Assistant Professor in the Division of Nutritional Sciences at Cornell University, where she provides leadership for the Cooperative Extension's maternal and child nutrition education program and conducts research in nutrition education. She is currently serving on the Board of Directors of the Society for Nutrition Education.

Martha Plass, M.S., is a Nutrition Education Specialist with Project NEAT (Nutrition Education Awareness and Training), a Nutrition Education and Training program serving four suburban Philadelphia counties.

Jill Randell, M.S., M.Ed., R.D., formerly at Cornell University, is a Nutrition Education Specialist with the Food and Nutrition Service, U.S. Department of Agriculture.

Allene G. Vaden, Ph.D., is Associate Professor of Dietetics, Restaurant, and Institutional Management, and scientist at Kansas Agricultural Experiment Station, Kansas State University. She is editor of the *School Food Service Research Review* and serves on the editorial policy councils of the *Journal of Nutrition Education* and the *Journal of Allied Health*.

INDEX